ADVANCES IN THE SCIENTIFIC EVALUATION OF BLADDER CANCER AND MOLECULAR BASIS FOR DIAGNOSIS AND TREATMENT

Edited by **Raj Persad**
and **Weranja Ranasinghe**

Advances in the Scientific Evaluation of Bladder Cancer and Molecular Basis for Diagnosis and Treatment

http://dx.doi.org/10.5772/56665

Edited by Raj Persad and Weranja Ranasinghe

Contributors

Yasuyoshi Miyata, Nan-Haw Chow, Hsiao-Sheng Liu, Martin Schumacher, Daisy Salvadori, Glenda Nicioli Da Silva, Weranja Ranasinghe, Raj Persad, Mariana Bisarro Dos Reis, Claudia Rainho

Published by InTech

Janeza Trdine 9, 51000 Rijeka, Croatia

Publishing Process Manager Sandra Bakic
Typesetting InTech DTP Team
Cover InTech Design Team

Additional hard copies can be obtained from orders@intechopen.com

Advances in the Scientific Evaluation of Bladder Cancer and Molecular Basis for Diagnosis and Treatment,
Edited by Raj Persad and Weranja Ranasinghe
p. cm.
ISBN 978-953-51-1142-9

For EU product safety concerns:
IN TECH d.o.o., Prolaz Marije Krucifikse Kozulić 3, 51000 Rijeka, Croatia,
info@intechopen.com or visit our website at intechopen.com.

Meet the editors

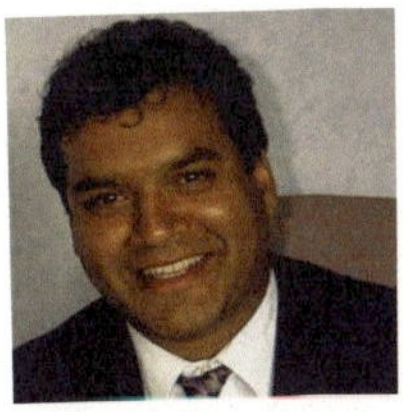

Professor Raj Persad has been a practising Uro-Oncology surgeon with an international reputation for innovation and research since 1996. He has served on key National steering committees for guideline development, service reform and research such as the NCIN, NCRI, NICE, NIHR, BAUS Section of Oncology and Cancer Research UK. He is one of the country's leading pelvic cancer surgeons with collaborations abroad in the US and Europe. He has been involved in drug discovery and development over the last 20 years as well as surgical device development. He has been Chief and Principle Investigator for a number of portfolio clinical trials. He has over 250 publications and received in excess of £4m in cancer research grants.

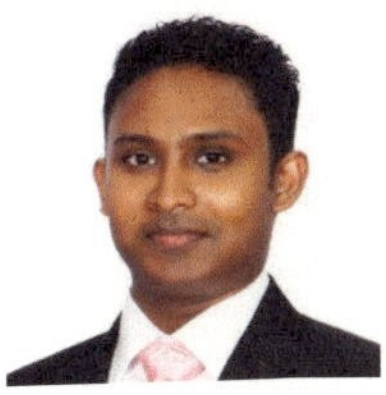

Mr. Weranja Ranasinghe is a urology trainee of the Royal Australiasian College of Surgeons and is currently enrolled in a PhD degree by the University of Melbourne at the Austin hospital, Australia. He graduated from the University of Bristol, UK in 2006 and was awarded the MRCS diploma by the Royal College of Surgeons Edinburgh, UK in 2008. His main interests are in prostate and other urological cancers. He has been principle researcher of a number of studies with international collaborations including the UK and the US resulting publications in peer reviewed journals and has received a number of awards and grants for his research.

Contents

Preface

Bladder cancer is the sixth most common cancer in the world affecting more than 300,000 men and women worldwide. The diagnosis of bladder cancer not only places a significant personal burden on individuals suffering with the disease (with regular need for surveillance and potential for surgery/radiotherapy) but also has a huge economic and psychosocial and psychosexual impact.

This book is a collection of articles by experts in the field of bladder cancer. It summarises the vast breadth of current knowledge of the molecular processes and the genetic and epigenetic modulation involved in bladder carcinogenesis of the bladder, carcinoma in-situ and the current treatment modalities of bladder cancer.

Tobacco smoking and also a number of occupational carcinogens have been linked to bladder cancer. However the mechanisms involved in the carcinogenesis process are complex and involve multiple steps. Thus, the mechanisms behind DNA damage, regulatory pathways and genetic and epi-genetic modulation leading to bladder carcinogenesis are discussed, highlighting the molecular targets of chemotherapy.

Focus has been placed on carcinoma-in situ of the bladder, an under emphasised but potentially aggressive and fatal form of pre-cancer which is increasing in incidence. Thus an overview of this condition discussing the epidemiology, risk factors, presentation and the management has been included.

Furthermore, this book also discusses the treatment of muscle invasive disease, immunotherapy and advances in molecular signalling pathways with future therapeutic potential. Therefore the roles of adjuvant and neo-adjuvent chemotherapy as well as other agents used in muscle invasive bladder cancer and immune therapy have been included.

We believe that this book will provide an excellent overview of the molecular mechanics underlying bladder carcinoma and their role in current and future therapy and would be integral for clinicians and researchers in the field of bladder cancer.

Editor:
Professor Raj Persad. MBBS, ChM, FRCS, FRCS (Urol), FEBU.
Spire Bristol Hospital, UK

Co-editor:
Mr. Weranja Ranasinghe MBChB, MRCSED.
Cabrini Hospital, Melbourne, Australia

Chapter 1

Genetic Instability in Normal-Appearing and Tumor Urothelium Cells and the Role of the TP53 Gene in the Toxicogenomic Effects of Antineoplastic Drugs

Daisy Maria Favero Salvadori and
Glenda Nicioli da Silva

Additional information is available at the end of the chapter

http://dx.doi.org/10.5772/53502

1. Introduction

Bladder cancer is one of the most common urinary neoplasms in industrialized countries, with more than 50,000 new cases diagnosed annually in Europe and North America [1,2]. In most countries of the Western world, transitional cell carcinomas (TCCs) account for 90% of the malignancies of this organ, while 5% are identified as squamous cell carcinomas and 2% as adenocarcinomas [3]. Approximately 80% of TCCs are low-grade tumors that are papillary, non-invasive and usually superficial, with stages Ta and Tis; the remaining 20% are high-grade papillary or non-papillary tumors that are often invasive or metastatic, with stages T1–T4. The five-year survival rate for TCC patients is 50%. The involvement of the bladder muscular wall signifies a worse prognosis and requires aggressive medical intervention such as radical cystectomy [4,5].

Occupational exposures in the textile and tire industries were the first factors implicated in the induction of bladder cancer. Currently, the prolonged use of phenacetin analgesics, exposure to cyclophosphamide, and smoking are the main risk factors associated with the etiology of transitional cell carcinoma [6]. Although men are 3-4 times more likely to develop bladder cancer, women present more often with advanced disease and have a lower probability of survival [7]. According to Shariat et al.[8], age is also considered a risk factor for urothelial carcinoma because the incidence of this cancer increases progressively with age; the incidence is higher after 60 years and peaks at 70 years, when the risk is 2% to 4% in men and 0.5% to 1% in women [9].

Clinically, the main problem associated with urothelial tumors is their highly unpredictable potential to progress to muscle-invasive disease, become multifocal and recur [5,10]. The recurrences might be *de novo* lesions that are different from recidivates, which occur because of incomplete resection of the primary tumor. After resection and/or treatment of a primary tumor, *de novo* TCC occurs in 50% to 70% of patients over a period of 4–5 years of follow-up. In fact, it has been suggested that patients undergoing surgical procedures are at a high risk for developing new neoplasia and are also susceptible to recurrences, possibly because of the presence of urothelial genetic instabilities [11-13].

Two hypotheses have been proposed to explain the association between urothelial carcinogenesis, multifocality and recurrence. The first hypothesis suggests a monoclonal origin of the lesions. In other words, multifocal or recurrent tumors originate from a single transformed cell that proliferates and colonizes other parts of the bladder through intraepithelial migration or transportation by urine. The second hypothesis proposes a polyclonal origin, suggesting that urine carcinogens that are in contact with multiple sites lead to the development of independent multifocal tumors [14,15]. The understanding of the clonality of multifocal bladder tumors is important to establish therapeutic strategies because new therapies often target specific molecules in these tumors [10].

2. DNA mutation and bladder carcinogenesis

Tumors are made up of billions of cells that originate from an initial cell that eluded apoptosis, accumulated genetic alterations and multiplied clonally [16]. It is expected that both external and internal factors contribute to these genetic mutations. External factors include lifestyle, such as excessive alcohol consumption, an unhealthy diet, exposure to excessive sunlight and chemical carcinogens, lack of exercise and smoking [17]. Internal factors include gene mutations, changes in the hormonal and immune systems, and metabolic abnormalities. During cell division, spontaneous genetic errors occur at an estimated frequency of approximately 10^{-5} to 10^{-6} [18]. Therefore, the blockade of apoptosis can favor the accumulation of mutated cells, a critical event in cancer pathogenesis [19].

Carcinogenesis is a multistep process that involves initiation, promotion and progression. Initiation is characterized by the formation of a preneoplastic cell resulting from an irreversible genotoxic event (gene mutation) caused by chemical, physical or biological carcinogens. This mutation usually occurs in genes that control the cell cycle, cell differentiation, apoptosis and DNA repair, leading to the survival of cells with genetic alterations [20]. The promotion stage involves the selective clonal expansion of the initiated cell through an increase in cell growth or a decrease in apoptosis, leading to an accumulation of mutations and an increase in the level of genetic instability (genetic and epigenetic changes) [20]. The third step, progression, involves genetic events such as changes in ploidy and chromosome integrity and results in a change from the preneoplastic state to the neoplastic state, producing cells with a high degree of anaplasia, an imbalance between cell proliferation and apoptosis and self-sufficiency (e.g., growth and multiplication independent of stimuli - Figure 1) [20,21].

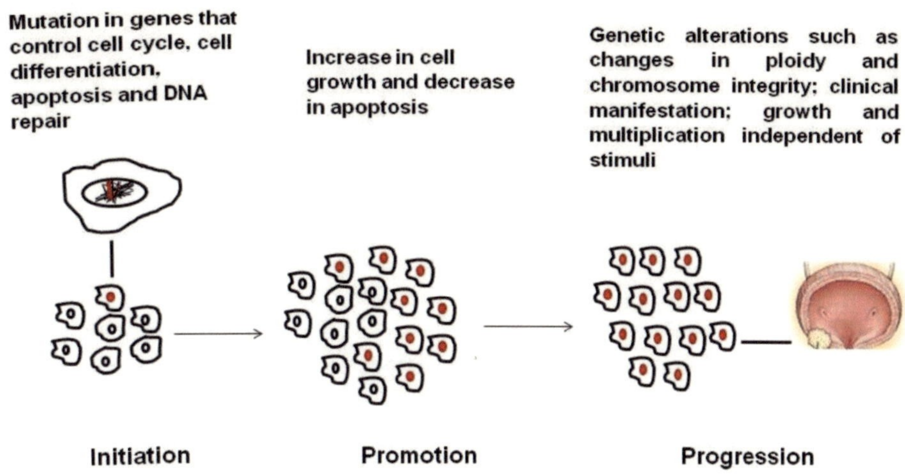

Figure 1. Multistep process of carcinogenesis

Urinary bladder carcinogenesis also occurs through multiple stages that are characterized by genetic changes that reflect the malignant transformation of an initiated normal cell [22]. These changes can occur in oncogenes/protooncogenes, tumor suppressor gene, regions of microsatellites, and cell cycle regulatory genes [23], which can trigger a framework of genetic instability characterized by a significant increase in the mutation rate (an early event in carcinogenesis). Genetic instability can be divided into two types: the first type comprises the insertions/deletions (basic single nucleotide changes) that result in read errors and are often observed in microsatellite regions (microsatellite instability), and the second type comprises the loss or gain of whole chromosomes or chromosome fragments (chromosomal changes), resulting in the loss or amplification of regions of DNA that contain genes crucial for neoplastic development [24].

Several studies have shown that many genetic and molecular alterations are involved in the initiation and progression stages of TCC, although the mechanisms responsible for the malignant phenotype are not completely understood. It is known that the accumulation of genetic changes, and not just a single mutation, determines the clinical behavior of TCC [25]. In fact, several studies have demonstrated the existence of numerous chromosomal changes in neoplastic and non-neoplasic urothelial cells from patients with a history of bladder cancer. The most frequent changes are polysomy of chromosomes 3, 7 and 17 and monosomy of chromosome 9 [26-30]. Furthermore, some authors have observed that 100% of patients with chromosome 17 loss exhibit recurrence [31]. Genetic analyses have also shown that the oncogenes *RAS* (related to recurrence), *erb-B2* (related to cell survival) and *EGF/EGFR* (related to recurrence and tumor progression) are the most important prognostic markers for bladder cancer [32]. Microsatellite alterations on chromosome 9 are indicative of genomic instability [33], but chromosome 9q segment loss (in low-grade papillary TCC), *FGFR3* mutations (low grade non-invasive tumors with low potential of progression) and the loss of *TP53* function (associated with muscle-invasive disease and metastatic potential) have also been described

[34,35]. Additionally, some authors have reported that *SOCS-1, STAT-1, BCL-2, DAPK,* and *E-cadherin* gene methylation are linked to tumor recurrence [36].

The *TP53* tumor suppressor gene has an important role in the cellular responses to various stress agents, including DNA damage [37,38]. After DNA damage occurs, *TP53* induces the transient or permanent blockage of cell proliferation or activates cell death signaling pathways [39]. However, it has been shown that some mutations in human tumors abolish or attenuate the binding of p53 protein to its consensus DNA sequence, abolishing the transcriptional activation of *TP53* target genes and resulting in the partial or complete loss of p53 function [40]. In fact, some studies have demonstrated that bladder tumor cells are grouped based on their molecular alterations in the *TP53* and *RB* signaling pathways [41]. Several mutations were found to confer new functions to mutant p53 that are independent of the wild-type p53 [42]. These findings have several implications, including a possible heterogeneous clinical phenotype depending on whether p53 itself is mutated and the site of the mutations or whether the p53 function is indirectly modified [43]. It has been demonstrated that genes related to cellular communication, cell cycle, cell division, cell death, cellular component organization, cell adhesion, and cell proliferation pathways, among others, are closely associated with the tumor grade. Although gene networks vary according to the tumor grade, *TP53* and several other genes have been frequently shown to be associated with the malignant phenotype of bladder tumors [44]. Independent of the *TP53* status, differences have been reported in several signaling pathways, such as the AMP kinase, JAK/STAT3, and MAP kinase (p38 MAPK, ERK, JNK) pathways. The downregulation of the *adipoR1* (involved in the AMP kinase pathway), *ABCA7* (involved in the ERK phosphorylation pathway), *DUSP22* (involved in the ERK and MAPK pathways), and *AKAP7* (involved in second messenger-mediated signaling events) genes was observed in cells with different tumor grades. Similarly, genes related to transcription, replication and DNA synthesis are also differentially expressed independent of the *TP53* status [44]. Additionally, no relationship between tumor grade or *TP53* status and the expression of *ANLN* and *S100P* (genes used as progression biomarkers in some types of tumors) in TCC lines has been described [44].

In normal cells, the p53 level is regulated by the interaction of the proteins mdm2, cop1, jnk and pirh2, which promote p53 degradation (ubiquitin/proteasome pathway) (Figure 2). After exposure to genotoxic or non-genotoxic stressors, the level of p53 is increased because the interaction with mdm2 and other regulators is inhibited. Then, several modulators (kinases, acetylases, etc) activate p53 transcriptional activity. The final result of p53 activation is either cell cycle arrest and DNA repair or apoptosis (Figure 3) [45].

Smoking is usually associated with the development of persistent clones of DNA-damaged cells in the urothelium and may partially explain the continuous occurrence of genetically aberrant cells in the mucosa. It is important to note that increased DNA damage has been detected in the transitional cells of smokers and ex-smokers who are free of neoplasia and have normal urinary bladder cell cytology [46]. Cytogenetic analyses have shown that bladder tumor recurrence is associated with high levels of DNA damage, which are still present in the normal-appearing urothelium of patients surgically treated for TCC [12]. Data suggest that part of this damage might occur through both clastogenic and aneugenic events, as detected by the micronucleus test (Figure 4) in TCC patients (J.P. Castro Marcondes personal communication, July 18, 2012). The increased level of DNA damage in cytologically "normal" cells from patients with a history of TCC has been shown to be related to the tumor histological grade, regardless of the length of time or clinical course since resection, suggesting these cells may be new TCC precursors or subclones of a previous TCC. Based on these data, it has been suggested that the primary tumor represents only the most obvious component of the disease, and several foci of secondary "reseeded" or "relocated" anomalous urothelium exist or may appear when the primary neoplasm is diagnosed [12]. Therefore, the genetic follow-up of patients after surgery must be a routine because elevated levels of DNA damage could predict recurrence.

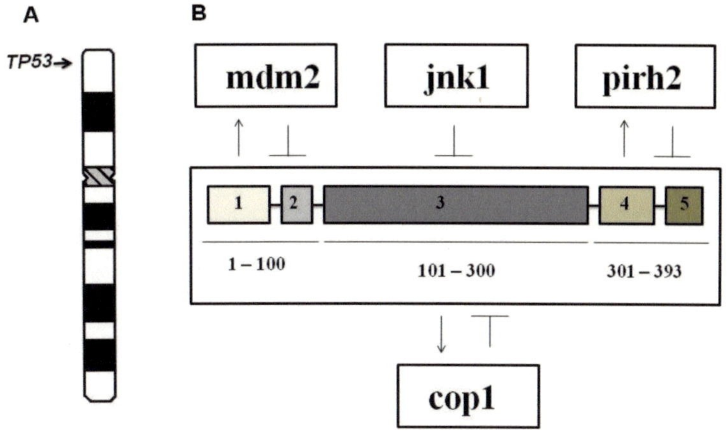

Figure 2. The *TP53* gene and the p53 protein. A) The *TP53 locus*: chromosome 17 (17p13.1); B) the p53 protein (1 - acidic transactivation domain and mdm2 protein binding site (amino-terminus), 2 – proline-rich region and second transactivation domain, 3 - DNA binding domain, 4 - oligomerization domain and 5 - non-specific DNA binding domain that binds to damaged DNA (carboxy-terminus)) and regulators. Adapted from [45].

Cystoscopy and cytology are considered standard procedures for monitoring patients with a history of TCC and individuals with bladder cancer symptoms (hematuria, pollakiuria and dysuria). However, these exams have a very limited ability to detect microscopic lesions and are subjective because they depend on the cytopathologist's experience; therefore, these tests have very low sensitivity for low-grade lesions [47]. It has been shown that only 61% of patients with biopsies positive for TCC had a similar diagnosis based on the cytological analysis [48]. On the other hand, some authors have reported 100% agreement between biopsies and cytogenetic analysis results using probes for the centromeres of chromosomes 3, 7 and 17 and the 9p21 locus. Thus, the use of techniques that increase the sensitivity and specificity of early TCC detection, both in patients undergoing bladder tumor resection and in patients considered at risk for TCC, must be taken into consideration. In this context, biomarkers linked to the behavior of a particular biological entity (e.g., chromosome damage) might be used to assess cancer risk in different tissues.

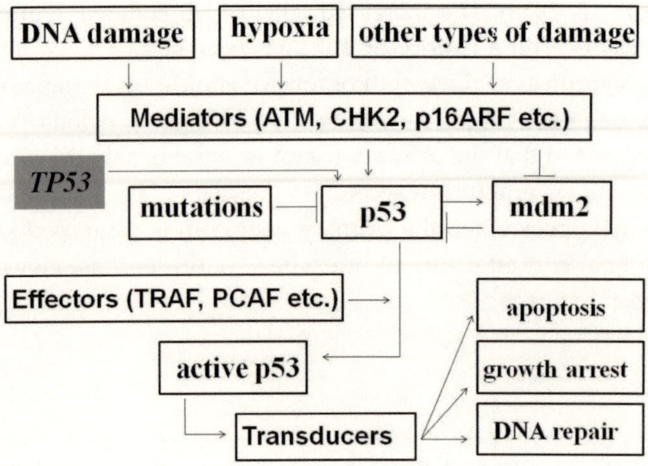

Figure 3. Upstream and downstream p53 activation pathways. Adapted from [45].

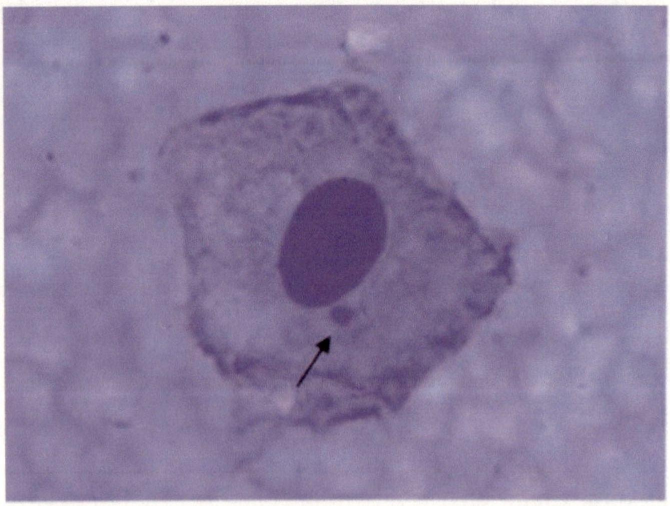

Figure 4. Exfoliated urothelial cell with a micronucleus (arrow). Giemsa stain (X 1000). Adapted from [49].

3. Bladder cancer and chemotherapy

It is import to know the disease stage to effectively plan the treatment for bladder cancer. Different types of treatments are available, including surgery, biologic therapy, radiotherapy, and chemotherapy. TCC has been efficiently treated with radiotherapy and combinations of different antineoplastic compounds. Intravesical Bacillus Calmette Guérin (BCG) instillations have shown success as adjuvant treatment for patients with intermediate and high risk non-muscle-invasive bladder tumor [50]. BCG induces a massive influx of cytokines and inflammatory cells into the bladder wall and lumen [51]. Moreover, BCG therapy has been demonstrated to reduce the recurrence rate and the risk of progression to muscle invasive disease in patients with carcinoma in situ and superficial bladder tumors [52].

Combined chemotherapy protocols have been extensively studied with the goal of improving bladder cancer treatment and the overall survival rate [53]. The standard protocol includes the drugs methotrexate, vinblastine, doxorubicin and cisplatin (MVAC) [54], but gemcitabine has also been successfully introduced [55]. The primary effect induced by these drugs is DNA damage with consequent cell cycle arrest and apoptosis. However, tumor cells have different levels of sensitivity to therapeutic agents, which may affect treatment success. Moreover, the genetic background of each tumor/patient must be taken into account to ensure treatment efficacy. In the context of developing chemotherapy protocols, the characterization of genes associated with a tumor's sensitivity to antitumor agents plays a critical role in the selection of the optimal treatment [56].

In 2000, Von der Maase et al. [54] demonstrated that the gemcitabine/cisplatin regimen had an efficacy similar to that of the MVAC protocol but with superior safety and tolerability, thus providing a potential standard alternative to treat bladder cancer. Gemcitabine is a deoxycytidine analog, which is phosphorylated to yield an active dFdCTP metabolite (gemcitabine triphosphate) that is incorporated into DNA, causing DNA strand breaks and thereby eliciting a DNA damage response characterized by cell cycle arrest in the G1/S phase and replication blockage [57,58]. Gemcitabine can also be incorporated into RNA to inhibit RNA synthesis [59]. Because of its low molecular weight of 299 Da, (lower than the molecular weights of drugs commonly used in intravesical chemotherapy; e.g., mitomycin C and doxorubicin), gemcitabine is able to penetrate the bladder mucosa, which has beneficial effects on the treatment of invasive bladder cancers [60]. Cisplatin is one of the most potent antitumor agents, with the ability to induce DNA crosslinking and apoptosis [61,62]. A molecule of cisplatin consists of a central atom of platinum surrounded by two chlorine atoms and two ammonia groups. Cisplatin is activated by the reaction of water molecules with the chloride ions. This activated compound than reacts with DNA, RNA, proteins and phospholipid membranes [63]. Similar to other platinum compounds, cisplatin forms DNA adducts between adjacent guanines (65%) and between guanine and adenine (25%) and forms interstrand crosslinks (10%) that interfere with DNA replication and repair, contributing to its antitumor efficacy [64,65].

The *TP53* status had been shown to play a pivotal role in the response to a large panel of anticancer drugs. Numerous studies have investigated the relationship between the tumor suppressor protein p53 and/or *TP53* gene mutations and the response to chemotherapy. Cote et al. [66] demonstrated that the presence of a normal functional *TP53* is associated with a good response to chemotherapy, and Hall et al. [67] suggested that the existence of *TP53* allelic variants indicates a complex role for the *TP53* pathway in human neoplasias. Therefore, differences among *TP53* responses may reflect the complex biology of this gene with respect to the regulation of apoptosis and cell proliferation. Because the *TP53* network is linked to many other cellular pathways, it is possible that defects in some of these pathways might qualitatively or quantitatively interfere with p53 function. Moreover, p53 is only one component of a giant surveillance network modulated by many other elements, including negative (Mdm2, Mdmx, Pirh2 and COP1) [68] and positive (DERP6) [69] regulators of p53, other members of the p53 family and several other signaling pathways [70].

The *TP53* and p53 status have also been used as biological markers to predict the response to chemotherapy. However, p53 expression and BCG response have shown contradictory results in literature. While some authors have concluded that p53 expression is not suitable as a marker to predict BCG response [71,72], other have stated that p53 has potential to be used as an independent marker to distinguish BCG responders and BCG non-responders in terms of time to recurrence and progression and progression to muscle invasive disease [73,74]. Moreover, independent on *TP53* status, some investigators have reported that the BCG therapy induces cellular reactive oxygen species and lipid peroxidation in cancer cells, inducing DNA damage, which could lead to mutations that select for their survival [75]. Thus, the authors suggest that reducing either the number of instillations of BCG that patients receive or the dose of BCG may reduce the amount of ROS and DNA damage and could lead to reduced disease progression [75]. Other authors have conclude that BCG response depend on the combination of markers to provide important information for selecting patients for the appropriate treatment [76].

On the other hand, there are few data in the literature regarding the relationship between this biomarker and the response to gemcitabine or cisplatin [77-80]. With regard to cell cycle kinetics, gemcitabine or combined treatment with gemcitabine plus cisplatin induces G1 cell cycle arrest in TCC cell lines *in vitro* independent of the *TP53* status. Conversely, only the cell responses to cisplatin were dependent on the *TP53* status. Whereas the wild-type *TP53* cells stopped in S phase, the *TP53*-mutated cells accumulated in G2 phase [81]. Similar findings have been described regarding apoptosis: whereas cisplatin induces apoptosis in only wt-*TP53* cells, apoptosis occurs in cells treated with gemcitabine or gemcitabine plus cisplatin independent of the *TP53* status, although higher percentages are observed in the wt-*TP53* cells [81]. In wt-*TP53* cells, gemcitabine-induced cellular damage can stimulate p53 expression, resulting in p21 expression and cell cycle arrest, enabling DNA damage repair or inducing apoptosis mediated by the *BAX* gene. In cells with a mutated *TP53* phenotype, the expression of p53 and p21 cannot be induced, but *BAX* can still be expressed, resulting in apoptosis [82]. Regarding cytotoxicity, *TP53*-wt cells were more resistant to cisplatin and more sensitive to gemcitabine than mutated *TP53* cells [81]. Some authors have suggested that the effect of cisplatin on human cancer cells has characteristics of senescence rather than apoptosis [83]. According to these authors, cancer cells lacking *TP53* function can also be killed via a TP53-independent mechanism, similar to replicative senescence. However, combined treatment with cisplatin and gemcitabine was more effective in reducing cell survival than treatment with the two drugs individually, independent of the *TP53* status [81]. Interestingly, genetic networks determined by Bayesian interpolation and built from microarray data show that, *in vitro*, TCC cell lines do not establish positive or negative relationships between *TP53* and a group of genes but instead exhibit direct interactions between *TP53* and many genes. Furthermore, different gene networks have been observed according to the tumor cell lines were obtained, confirming that other genes and pathways are involved in the chemotherapy response, independent of the TP53 status [44]. It is known that both gemcitabine and cisplatin act by inducing DNA structural damage and modulating gene expression. Some authors have demonstrated that gemcitabine has cytotoxic and genotoxic effects in murine bone marrow [84], and other authors have confirmed the genotoxic effect of antineoplastic drugs in circulating blood lymphocytes [85]. Several studies revealed that cisplatin is an effective clastogen and inducer of both sister chromatid exchange and micronuclei development [86,87]. Furthermore, several authors have demonstrated that cisplatin induces a noticeable mutagenic effect, increasing the frequency of micronuclei and the percentage of chromosome aberrations in rat bone-marrow cells [88]. Additionally, Brozovic et al. [89] reported that cisplatin induces strong genotoxicity in murine peripheral blood leucocytes and brain, liver and kidney cells. In bladder cancer cells, gemcitabine and cisplatin, alone or in combination, have been shown to cause significant DNA damage at different tumor development stages independent of the *TP53* status (Figure 5). However, *TP53*-mutated TCC cells are more resistant to the genotoxic effects induced by the combined treatment with gemcitabine and cisplatin than wild-type cells are (E.A de Carmargo personal communication, June 27, 2012). Regarding the toxicogenomic and proteomics events, Nordentoft et al. [90] demonstrated that the relationship between the transcription factor TFAP2α and cisplatin or gemcitabine sensitivity in bladder cancer cells is dependent on p53 because TFAP2α silencing increased the proliferation of only the wild type *TP53* bladder cells and reduced cisplatin- and gemcitabine-induced cell death. Additionally, Gazzaniga et al [91] reported that gemcitabine induces apoptosis in *TP53*-mutated cells, involving caspase-3, -8 and -9 activation but no changes in *Bcl-2, Bax, survivin* and *Bcl-X* expression. In fact, the gemcitabine-induced modulation of *Bax* expression has been observed only in a wild-type *TP53* cell line (Da Silva et al., 2012, unpublished data, [92]). In contrast, following treatment with gemcitabine or cisplatin plus gemcitabine, there was an observable upregulation of the *GADD45A* and *CDKN1A* genes independent of the *TP53* status in bladder cancer cell lines, thus providing possible links to apoptosis and cell cycle arrest (Da Silva et al., 2012, unpublished data). On the other hand, Cho et al [93] reported that *Bcl-2* upregulation in a *TP53* mutated bladder cancer cell line contributes to the development of cisplatin resistance, and targeting this gene with an siRNA may therefore be a potential tool to reverse cisplatin resistance. Matsui et al [94] also reported that the expression of the galectin-7 gene could serve as a candidate predictive marker for chemosensitivity to cisplatin in wild-type *TP53* cells.

In conclusion, while there is evidence implicating the role of *TP53* in the regulation of DNA repair and apoptosis and as a molecular node, other target genes can also be modulated by antineoplastic compounds and influence the success of drug therapy. Regardless of tumor-associated *TP53* mutations or the tumor grade, simultaneous treatment with cisplatin and gemcitabine is an effective protocol for transitional cell carcinomas. In this context, because high concentrations of cisplatin are toxic to humans, the use of low concentrations of cisplatin and gemcitabine in combination might be clinically relevant in reducing the secondary effects of chemotherapy [81].

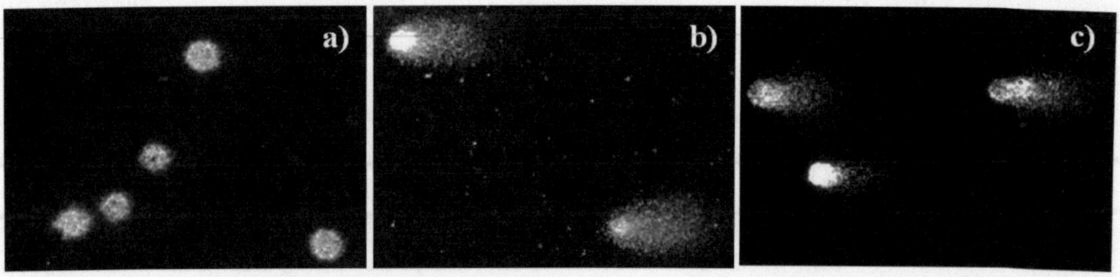

Figure 5. Genotoxic damage induced by cisplatin and gemcitabine in transitional carcinoma cells, as depicted by the comet assay. (A) Untreated cells; (B) cells treated with cisplatin; (C) cells treated with gemcitabine. Ethidium bromide staining (X 400).

4. Actual scenario

Most cellular components exert their functions by interacting with other components located within the same cell, in different cells, or even in different organs. In humans, the complexity of the interaction networks (the human interactome) is impressive: there are approximately 25,000 protein-coding genes, approximately 1,000 metabolites and an indefinite number of distinct proteins and functional RNA molecules. Therefore, the number of cellular components capable of being regulatory interactome centers exceeds 100000 [95]. Moreover, the intra- and inter-cellular connectivity implies that the impact of genetic abnormality is not restricted to the activity of the gene product but can have effects on other genes and their products that might have no defect. Several authors have suggested that the disease phenotype is rarely a consequence of abnormalities in a single gene product but reflects various patho-biological processes that interact in a complex network [96]. Therefore, the effects of cell interconnection on disease progression can lead to the identification of genes and systems that offer better targets for drug development. Moreover, the potential use of microRNA in the future therapeutic interventions has also been discussed. For example, the effects of miR-100 on cell growth and clonogenic capacity in TCC cell lines emphasize a possible link between this miRNA and bladder carcinoma pathogenesis [97]. These new concepts may identify more accurate biomarkers for monitoring the functional integrity of networks and classifying diseases [96].

Changes in gene expression profiles may be immediate and more sensitive markers of drug toxicity than markers that are typically analyzed in toxicity tests (morphological changes, carcinogenicity and reproductive markers) [98]. Furthermore, some authors have shown that the implementation of proteomic platforms for the identification of novel targets of interest (membrane antigens, protein overexpression, etc.) is gaining widespread attention. The incorporation of biomarkers in clinical proteomics studies has also become important to define biologically effective therapeutic protocols for each patient and type of disease [99]. Thus, studies comparing gene and protein expression can confirm and emphasize the importance of using different technologies to understand and characterize complex biological systems.

5. Final conclusion

In this chapter, we presented data that demonstrate that high levels of DNA damage in normal-appearing urothelium are associated with tumor recurrence in patients treated for bladder TCC. Furthermore, the identification of genes associated with the sensitivity of tumors to chemotherapeutic drugs may play an important role in selecting the most efficient treatment protocol. Therefore, biomarker identification is relevant not only for diagnostic accuracy and prognosis but also for cancer therapy.

Currently, the ability of genomics and proteomics techniques to identify biomarkers and increase our understanding of complex cellular networks has been demonstrated. Thus, high-throughput methodologies help characterize diseases and increase our understanding of tumor progression mechanisms and the chemotherapy results. It is known that the primary effects of antineoplastic drugs are linked to DNA damage, leading to molecular events that may result in cell cycle arrest and apoptosis, which are essential responses for the maintenance of genetic integrity and cell viability [100]. Furthermore, it is known that early detection and treatment result in better survival rates for patients without clinical symptoms during the early stages of carcinogenesis [101].

Abbreviations

BCG – Baccillus Calmette Guérin

TCC – Transitional cell carcinoma

MVAC - Methotrexate, Vinblastine, Doxorubicin and Cisplatin

Author details

Daisy Maria Favero Salvadori* and Glenda Nicioli da Silva

*Address all correspondence to: dfavero@fmb.unesp.br

UNESP – Universidade Estadual Paulista; Botucatu Medical School; Department Pathology, Botucatu, Brazil

References

[1] Frau DV, Usai P, Dettori T, Caria P, De Lisa A, Vanni R. Fluorescence in situ hybridization patterns in newly diagnosed superficial bladder lesions and corresponding bladder washings. Cancer Genetics and Cytogenetics 2006;169(1) 21–26.

[2] Shelley MD, Mason MD, Kynaston H. Intravesical therapy for superficial bladder cancer: a systematic review of randomised trials and meta-analyses. Cancer Treatment Reviews 2010;36(6) 195-205.

[3] Cordon-Cardo C. Molecular alterations associated with bladder cancer initiation and progression. Scandinavian Journal of Urology and Nephrology 2008;218 154-165.

[4] Kaufman DS. Challenges in the treatment of bladder cancer. Annual Oncology 2006;17(5) 106-112.

[5] Castillo-Martin M, Domingo-Domenech J, Karni-Schmidt O, Matos T, Cordon-Cardo C. Molecular pathways of urothelial development and bladder tumorigenesis. Urology Oncology 2010;28(4) 401–408.

[6] Wallerand H, Bakkar AA, Diez de Medina SG, Pairon JC, Yang YC, Vordos D. Mutations in TP53, but not FGFR3, in urothelial cell carcinoma of the bladder are influenced by smoking: contribution of exogenous versus endogenous carcinogens. Carcinogenesis 2005; 26(1) 177-184.

[7] Fajkovic H, Halpern JA, Cha EK, Bahadori A, Chromecki TF, Karakiewicz PI, Breinl E, Merseburger AS, Shariat SF. Impact of gender on bladder cancer incidence, staging, and prognosis. World Journal of Urology 2011;29(4) 457-463.

[8] Shariat SF, Milowsky S, Droller MJ, M.D. Bladder cancer in the elderly. Urology Oncology 2009;27 653–667.

[9] Kirkali Z, Chan T, Manoharan M, Algaba F, Bush C, Cheng L, et al. Bladder Cancer: Epidemiology, staging and grading, and diagnosis. Urology 2005;66(6):4-34.

[10] Denzinger S, Mohren K, Knuechel R, Wild PJ, Burger M, Wieland WF,Hartmann A, Stoehr R. Improved clonality analysis of multifocal bladder tumors by combination of histopathologic organ mapping, loss of heterozygosity, fluorescence in situ hybridization, and p53 analyses. Human pathology 2006;37(2) 143-157.

[11] Nilsson S, Ragnhammar P, Nygren P, Glimelius B. A Systematic Overview of chemotherapy effects in urothelial bladder cancer. Acta oncologic 2001;40(2-3) 371-390.

[12] Gontijo AM, Marcondes JPC, Elias FN, de Oliveira MLCS, Lima ROA, Salvadori DMF, Camargo JLV. DNA Damage in Cytologically Normal Urothelial Cells of Patients With a History of Urothelial Cell Carcinoma. Environmental and Molecular Mutagenesis 2002;40(3) 190–199.

[13] Latini DM, Lerner SP, Wade SW, Lee DW, Quale DZ. Bladder cancer detection, treatment and outcomes: opportunities and challenges. Urology 2010;75(2) 334–339.

[14] Hafner C, Knuechel R, Stoehr R, Hartmann A. Clonality of multifocal urothelial carcinomas: 10 years of molecular genetic studies. International Journal of Cancer 2002;101(1) 1-6.

[15] Paiss T, Wöhr G, Hautmann RE, Mattfeldt T, Müller M, Haeussler J, Vogel W. Some tumors of the bladder are polyclonal in origin. Journal of Urology 2002;167(2 Pt 1) 718-723.

[16] Trosko JE. Commentary: is the concept of "tumor promotion" a useful paradigm? Molecular Carcinogenesis 2001;30(3) 131– 137.

[17] Sankpal UT, Pius H, Khan M, Shukoor MI, Maliakal P,. Lee CM, Abdelrahim M, Connelly SF, & Riyaz Basha. Environmental factors in causing human cancers: emphasis on tumorigenesis. Tumor Biology 2012. [Epub ahead of print]

[18] Cohen SM, Lawsonta TA. Rodent bladder tumors do not always predict for humans. Cancer Letters 1995;93(1) 9–16.

[19] Qu W, Bortner CD, Sakurai T, Hobson MJ, Waalkes MP. Acquisition of apoptotic resistance in arsenic-induced malignant transformation: role of the JNK signal transduction pathway. Carcinogenesis 2002;23(1) 151–159.

[20] Vicent TL, Gatenby RA. An evolutionary model for initiation, promotion, and progression in carcinogenesis. International Journal of Oncology 2008;32(4) 729-737.

[21] Pitot, HC. Adventures in hepatocarcinogenesis. Annual Reviews of Pathology 2007;2 1-29.

[22] Philips JL, Richardson IC. Aneuploidy in bladder cancers: the utility of fluorescent in situ hybridization in clinical practice. BJU International 2006, 98(1) 33-37.

[23] Habuchi T, Marberger M, Droller MJ, Hemstreet III GP, Grossman HB, Schalken JA, et al. Prognostic markers for bladder cancer: international consensus panel on bladder tumor markers. Journal of Urology 2005;66(6A) 64-74.

[24] Catto JWF, Meuth M, Hamdy FC. Genetic instability and transitional cell carcinoma of the bladder. BJU International 2004;93(1) 19-24.

[25] Kim IY, Kim SJ. Role of bone morphogenetic proteins in transitional cell carcinoma cells. Cancer Letters 2006;241(1) 118-123.

[26] Kruger S, Mess F, Bohle A, Feller AC. Numerical aberrations of chromosome 17 and the 9p21 locus are independent predictors of tumor recurrence in non-invasive transitiona cell carcinoma of the urinary bladder. International Journal of Oncology 2003;23(1): 41-48.

[27] Obermann EC, Meyer S, Hellge D, Zaak D, Filbeck T, Stoehr R, Hofstaedter F, Hartmann A, Knuechel R. Fluorescence in situ hybridization detects frequent chromo-

some 9 deletions and aneuploidy in histologically normal urothelium of bladder cancer patients. Oncology Reports 2004;11(4): 745-751.

[28] Latif Z, Watters AD, Dunn I, Grigor K, Underwood MA, Bartlett JM. HER2/neu gene amplification and protein overexpression in G3 pT2 transitional cell carcinoma of the bladder: a role for anti-HER2 therapy? European Journal of Cancer 2004;4(1) 56-63.

[29] Degtar P, Neulander E, Zirkin H, Yusim I, Douvdevani A, Mermershtain W et al. Fluorescence in situ hybridization performed on exfoliated urothelial cells in patients with transitional cell carcinoma of the bladder. Urology 2004;63(2) 398-401.

[30] Pycha A, Lodde M, Comploj E, Negri G, Egarter-Vigl E, Vittadello F et al. Intermediate-risk urothelial carcinoma: na unresolved problem? Urology 2004;63(3) 472-475.

[31] Ishiwata S, Takahashi S, Homma Y, Tanaka Y, Kameyama S, Hosaka Y, Kitamura T. Nonivansive detection and prediction of bladder cancer by fluorescence in situ hybridization analysis of exfoliated urothelial cells in voided urine. Urology 2001;57(4) 811-815.

[32] Kausch I, Bohle A. Molecular aspects of bladder cancer III. Prognostic markers of bladder cancer. European Urology 2002;41(1) 15-29.

[33] Turyn J, Matuszewski M, Schlichtholz B. Genomic instability analysis of urine sediment versus tumor tissue in transitional cell carcinoma of the urinary bladder. Oncology Reports 2006;15(1) 259-265.

[34] Baithun Si, Naase M, Blanes A, Diaz-Cano Sj. Molecular and kinetic features of transitional cell carcinomas of the bladder: biological and clinical implications. Virchows Archives 2001;438(3) 289-297.

[35] Cheng L, Zhang S, MacLennan GT, Williamson SR, Lopez-Beltrn, Montironi R, FRCPath, IFCAP. Bladder cancer: translating molecular genetic insights into clinical practice. Human Pathology 2011;42(4) 455-481.

[36] Friedrich MG, Chandrasoma S, Siegmund KD, Cheng JC, Toma MI. Prognostic relevance of methylation markers in patients with non-muscle invasive bladder carcinoma. European Journal of Cancer 2005;41(17) 1009-1015.

[37] Kosmider B, Osiecka R, Zyner E, Ochocki J. Comparison between the genotoxicity of cis′Pt(II) complex of 3-aminoflavone and cis-DDP in lymphocytes evaluated by the comet assay. Drug and Chemical Toxicology 2005;28(2) 231-244.

[38] Basu A, Krishnamurthy S. Cellular Responses to Cisplatin-Induced DNA Damage. Journal of Nucleic Acids 2010, pii: 201367.

[39] Kim HG, Lee S, Kim DY, Ryu SY, Joo JK, Kim JC, Lee KH, Lee JH. Aberrant methylation of DNA Mismatch repair genes in elderly patients with sporadic gastric carcinoma: a comparision with younger patients. Journal of Surical Oncology 2010;101(1) 28-35.

[40] Kato S. Understanding the function structure and function mutation relationships of p53 tumor suppressor protein by high resolution missense mutation analysis. Proceedings of the National Academy of Sciences USA 2003;100(14) 8424–8429.

[41] Sanchez-Carbayo M, Socci ND, Charytonowicz E, Lu M, Prystowsky M, Childs G, Cordon-Cardo C. Molecular profiling of bladder cancer using cDNA microarrays: defining histogenesis and biological phenotypes. Cancer Research 2002;62(23) 6973–6980.

[42] Brosh R, Rotter V. When mutations gain new powers: news from the mutant p53 field. Nature Review Cancer 2009;9(10) 701–713.

[43] Prives C, Manfredi JJ. The continuing saga of p53—More sleepless nighs ahead. Molecular Cell 2005;19(6) 719–721.

[44] da Silva GN, Evangelista AF, Magalhães DA, Macedo C, Búfalo MC, Sakamoto-Hojo ET, Passos GA, Salvadori DM. Expression of genes related to apoptosis, cell cycle and signaling pathways are independent of TP53 status in urinary bladder cancer cells. Molecular Biology Reports 2011;38(6) 4159-4170.

[45] The TP53 website: http://p53.free.fr/index.html (accessed 20 July 2012).

[46] Gontijo AM, Elias FN, Salvadori DM, de Oliveira ML, Correa LA, Goldberg J, Trindade JC, de Camargo JL. Single-Cell Gel (Comet) Assay Detects Primary DNA Damage in Nonneoplastic Urothelial Cells of Smokers and Ex-smokers. Cancer Epidemiology, Biomarkers & Prevention 2001;10(9) 987-993.

[47] Fracasso ME, Franceschettia P, Doriaa D, Talaminib G, Bonettic F. DNA breaks as measured by the alkaline comet assay in exfoliated cells as compared to voided urine cytology in the diagnosis of bladder cancer: a study of 105 subjects. Mutation Research 2004;564(1) 57-64.

[48] Daniely M, Rona R, Kaplan T, Olsfanger S, Elboim L, Zilberstien Y et al. Combined analysis of morphology and fluorescence in situ hybridization significantly increases accuracy of bladder cancer detection in voided urine samples. Urology 2005;66(6) 1354-1359.

[49] Marcondes JPC. Cytogentic damage in exfoliated urothelial cell from patients with history of bladder transitional cell carcinoma. PhD thesis. Universidade Estadual Paulista; 2007.

[50] Babjuk M, OosterlinckW, Sylvester R, Kaasinen E, Böhle A, Palou-Redorta J, European Association of Urology (EAU). EAU guidelines on nonmuscle-invasive urothelial carcinoma of the bladder. European Urology 2008;54(2) 303–314.

[51] Kresowik TP, Griffith TS. Bacillus Calmette–Guerin immunotherapy for urothelial carcinoma of the bladder. Immunotherapy 2009;1(2) 281–288.

[52] Sylvester RJ, van der Meijden AP, Witjes JA, Kurth K. Bacillus Calmette–Guerin versus chemotherapy for the intravesical treatment of patients with carcinoma in situ of

the bladder: a meta-analysis of the published results of randomized clinical trials. Journal of Urology 2005;174(1) 86–91.

[53] Gallagher DJ, Milowsky MI, Bajorin DF. Advanced Bladder Cancer: Status of First-line Chemotherapy and the Search for Active Agents in the Second-line Setting. Cancer 2008; 113(6) 1284–1293.

[54] von der Maase H, Hansen SW, Roberts JT, Dogliotti L, Oliver T, Moore MJ, Bodrogi I, Albers P, Knuth A, Lippert CM, Kerbrat P, Sanchez Rovira P, Wersall P, Cleall SP, Roychowdhury DF, Tomlin I, Visseren-Grul CM, Conte PF. Gemcitabine and cisplatin versus methotrexate, vinblastine, doxorubicin and cisplatin in advanced or metastatic bladder cancer: Results of a large, randomized, multinational, multicenter, phase III study. Journal of Clinical Oncology 2000;18(17) 3068-3077.

[55] Bellmut J, Albiol S, Ramirez de Olano A, Pujadas J, Maroto P. On behalf the Spanish Oncology Genitourinary Group (SOGUG). Gemcitabine in the treatment of advanced transitional cell carcinoma of the urothelium. Annual Oncology 2006;17 113–117.

[56] Fujita H, Ohuchida K, Mizumoto K, Itaba S, Ito T, Nakata K, Yu J, Kayashima T, Souzaki R. Tajiri T, Manabe T, Ohtsuka T, Tanaka M. Gene expression levels as predictive markers of outcome in pancreatic cancer after gemcitabine-based adjuvant chemoterapy. Neoplasia 2010;12(10) 807-817.

[57] Galmarini CM, Clarke ML, Falette N, Puisieux A, Mackey JR, Dumontet C. Expression of a non-functional p53 affects the sensitivity of cancer cells to gemcitabine. International Journal of Cancer 2002;97(4) 439-445.

[58] Toschi L, Finocchiaro G, Gioia V. Role of gemcitabine in cancer therapy. Future Oncology 2005;1 7-17.

[59] Ruiz Van Haperen VWT, Veerman G, Vermoken JB, Peters GJ. 2',2'-Difluoro-deoxycytidine (gemcitabine) incorporation into RNA and DNA from tumor cell lines. Biochemical Pharmacology 1993;46(4) 762-766.

[60] Gontero P, Frea B. Actual experience and future development of gemcitabine in superficial bladder cancer. Annual Oncology 2006;17(5) 123-128.

[61] Wang D, Lippard SJ. Cellular processing of platinum anticancer drugs. Nature Reviews 2005;4(4) 307-319.

[62] Shimabukuro F, Neto CF, Sanches Jr J.A, Gattás GJF. DNA damage and repair in leukocytes of melanoma patients exposed in vitro to cisplatin. Melanoma Research 2011;21(2) 99-105.

[63] Cho JM, Manandhar S, Lee HR, Park HM, Kwak MK. Role of the Nrf2- antioxidant system in cytotoxicity mediated by anticancer cisplatin: Implication to cancer cell resistance. Cancer Letters 2008;260(1-2) 96–108.

[64] Rabik CA, Dolan ME. Molecular mechanisms of resistance and toxicity associated with platinating agents. Cancer Treatment Review 2007;33(1) 9–23.

[65] Stadler WM, Lerner SP, Groshen S, Stein JP, Shi SR, Raghavan D, Esrig D, Steinberg G, Wood D, Klotz L, Hall C, Skinner DG, Cote RJ. Phase III study of molecularly targeted adjuvant therapy in locally advanced urothelial cancer of the bladder based on p53 status. Journal of Clinical Oncology 2011;29(25) 3443-3449.

[66] Cote RJ, Esrig D, Groshen S, Jones PA, Skinne DG. P53 and treatment of bladder cancer. Nature 1997;385 124-125.

[67] Hall PA, McCluggage WG. Assessing p53 in clinical contexts: unlearned lessons and new perspectives. Journal of Pathoogy 2006;208(1) 1-6.

[68] Wang L, He G, Zhang P, Wang X, Jiang M, Yu L. Interplay between MDM2, MDMX, Pirh2 and COP1: the negative regulators of p53. Molecular Biology Reports 2010;38(1) 229-236.

[69] Yuan J, Tang W, Luo K, Chen X, Gu X, Wan B, Yu. Cloning and characterization of the human gene DERP6, which activates transcriptional activities of p53. Molecular Biology Reports 2006;33(3) 151–158.

[70] Soussi T, Wiman KG. Shaping genetic alterations in human cancer: the p53 mutation paradigm. Cancer Cell 2007;12(4) 303–312.

[71] Esuvaranathan K, Chiong E, Thamboo TP, Chan YH, Kamaraj R, Mahendran R, Teh M. Predictive value of p53 and pRb expression in superficial bladder cancer patients treated with BCG and interferon-alpha. Cancer 2007;109(6) 1097–1105.

[72] Peyromaure M, Weibing S, Sebe P, Verpillat P, Toublanc M, Dauge MC, Boccon-Gibod L, Ravery V. Prognostic value of p53 overexpression in T1G3 bladder tumors treated with bacillus Calmette-Guérin therapy. Urology 2002;59(3) 409–413.

[73] Saint F, Le Frere Belda MA, Quintela R, Hoznek A, Patard JJ, Bellot J, Popov Z, Zafrani ES, Abbou CC, Chopin DK, de Medina SG. Pretreatment p53 nuclear overexpression as a prognostic marker in superficial bladder cancer treated with bacillus Calmette–Guérin (BCG). European Urology 2004;45(4) 475–482.

[74] Palou J, Algaba F, Vera I, Rodriguez O, Villavicencio H, Sanchez-Carbayo M. Protein expression patterns of ezrin are predictors of progression in T1G3 bladder tumours treated with nonmaintenance bacillus Calmette-Guérin. European Urology 2009;56(5) 829–36.

[75] Rahmat JN, Esuvaranathan K, Mahendran R. Bacillus Calmette-Guérin induces cellular reactive oxygen species and lipid peroxidation in cancer cells. Urology 2012; 79(6) 1411.e15-20.

[76] Zuiverloon TC, Nieuweboer AJ, Vékony H, Kirkels WJ, Bangma CH, Zwarthoff EC. Markers predicting response to bacillus Calmette-Guérin immunotherapy in high-

risk bladder cancer patients: a systematic review. European Urology 2012;61(1) 128-145.

[77] Kielb SJ, Nikhil LS, Rubin MA, Sanda MG. Functional p53 mutation as a molecular determinant of paclitaxel and gemcitabine susceptibility in human bladder cancer. Journal of Urology 2001;166(2) 482–487.

[78] Fechner G, Perabo FGE, Schmidt DH, Haase L, Ludwig E, Schueller H, Blatter J, Muller C, Albers P. Prelinical evaluation of a radiosensitizingeffect of gemcitabine in p53 mutant and p53 wild type bladder cancer cells. Urology 2003;61(2) 468–473.

[79] Cory AH, Cory JG. Gemcitabine-induced apoptosis in a drug-resistant mouse leukemia L1210 cell line that does not express p53. Advances in Enzyme Regulation 2004;44 11–25.

[80] Yip HT, Chopra R, Chkrabarti R, Veena MS, Ramamurthy B, Srivatsan ES, Wang MB. Cisplatin-induced growth arrest of head and neck cancer cells correlates with increased expression of p16 and p53. Archives of Otolaryngology – Head & Neck Surgery 2006;132 (3) 317–26.

[81] da Silva GN, de Castro Marcondes JP, de Camargo EA, da Silva Passos Júnior GA, Sakamoto-Hojo ET, Salvadori DM. Cell cycle arrest and apoptosis in TP53 subtypes of bladder carcinoma cell lines treated with cisplatin and gemcitabine. Experimental Biology and Medicine (Maywood) 2010;235(7) 814-824.

[82] Bergman AM, Pinedo HM, Peters GJ. Determinants of resistance to 2′,2′- difluorodeoxycytidine (gemcitabine). Drug Resistance Updates 2002;5(1) 19-33.

[83] Wang X, Wong SC, Pan J, Tsao SW, Fung KH, Kwong DL, Sham JS, Nicholls JM. Evidence of cisplatin-induced senescent-like growth arrest in nasopharyngeal carcinoma cells. Cancer Research 1998;58(22) 5019–5022.

[84] Aydemir N, Bilaloğlu R. Genotoxicity of two anticancer drugs, gemcitabine and topotecan in mouse bone marrow in vivo. Mutation Research 2003;537(1) 43-51.

[85] Cavallo D, Ursini CL, Perniconi B, Francesco AD, Giglio M, Rubino FM, Marinaccio A, Iavicoli S. Evaluation of genotoxic effects induced by exposure to antineoplastic drugs in lymphocytes and exfoliated buccal cells of oncology nurses and pharmacy employees. Mutation Research 2005;10:587(1-2) 45-51.

[86] Choudhury RC, Jagdale MB, Misra S. Cytogenetic toxicity of cisplatin in bone marrow cells of Swiss mice. Journal of Chemotherapy 2000;12(2) 173-182.

[87] Kosmider B, Wyszynska K, Janik-Spiechowicz E, Osiecka R, Zyner E, Ochocki J, Ciesielska E, Wasowicz W. Evaluation of the genotoxicity of cis-bis(3-aminoflavone)dichloroplatinum(II) in comparison with cis-DDP. Mutation Research 2004; 14:558(1-2) 93-110.

[88] Rjiba-Touati K, Ayed-Boussema I, Skhiri H, Belarbia A, Zellema D, Achour A, Bacha H. Induction of DNA fragmentation, chromosome aberrations and micronuclei by

cisplatin in rat bone-marrow cells: Protective effect of recombinant human erythropoietin. Mutation Research. 2012;747(2) 202-206.

[89] Brozovic G, Orsolic N, Knezevic F, Horvat Knezevic A, Benkovic V, Sakic K, Borojevic N, Dikic D. The in vivo genotoxicity of cisplatin, isoflurane and halothane evaluated by alkaline comet assay in Swiss albino mice. Journal of Applied Genetics 2011;52(3) 355-361.

[90] Nordentoft I, Dyrskjøt L, Bødker JS, Wild PJ, Hartmann A, Bertz S, Lehmann J, Orntoft TF, Birkenkamp-Demtroder K. Increased expression of transcription factor TFAP2α correlates with chemosensitivity in advanced bladder cancer. BMC Cancer. 2011;11 135. PubMed PMID: 21489314

[91] Gazzaniga P, Silvestri I, Gradilone A, Scarpa S, Morrone S, Gandini O, Gianni W, Frati L, Aglianò AM. Gemcitabine-induced apoptosis in 5637 cell line: an in-vitro model for high-risk superficial bladder cancer. Anticancer Drugs 2007;18(2) 179-85.

[92] Da Silva GN, Camargo EA, Salvadori DMF. Toxicogenomic activity of gemcitabine in two TP53-mutated bladder cancer cell lines: special focus on cell cycle-related genes. Molecular Biology Reports 2012; DOI 10.1007/s11033-012-1916-1.

[93] Cho HJ, Kim JK, Kim KD, Yoon HK, Cho MY, Park YP, Jeon JH, Lee ES, Byun SS, Lim HM, Song EY, Lim JS, Yoon DY, Lee HG, Choe YK. Upregulation of Bcl-2 is associated with cisplatin-resistance via inhibition of Bax translocation in human bladder cancer cells. Cancer Letters 2006;237(1) 56-66.

[94] Matsui Y, Ueda S, Watanabe J, Kuwabara I, Ogawa O, Nishiyama H. Sensitizing effect of galectin-7 in urothelial cancer to cisplatin through the accumulation of intracellular reactive oxygen species. Cancer Research 2007;67(3) 1212-1220.

[95] Zhao Y, Jensen ON. Modification-specific proteomics: strategies for characterization of post-translational modifications using enrichments techniques. Proteomics 2009;9(20) 4632-4641.

[96] Barabasi A-L, Gulbahce N, Loscalo J. Network medicine: a network-based approach to human disease. Nature Reviews 2011;12(1) 56-68.

[97] Oliveira JC, Brassesco MS, Morales AG, Pezuk JA, Fedatto PF, da Silva GN, Srideli CA, Tone LG. MicroRNA-100 Acts as a Tumor Suppressor in Human Bladder Carcinoma 5637 Cells. Asian Pacific Journal of Cancer Prevention 2011;12(11) 3001-3004.

[98] Lee K-M, Kim J-H, Kang D. Design issues in toxicogenomics using DNA microarray experiment. Toxicology and Applied Pharmacology 2005;207(2) 200-208.

[99] Lee J-M, Han JJ, Altwerger G, Kohn EC. Proteomics and biomarkers in clinical trials for drug development. Journal of Proteomics 2011;74(12) 2632-2641.

[100] Tannock IF, Lee C. Evidence against apoptosis as a major mechanism for reproductive cell death following treatment of cell lines with anti-cancer drugs. British Journal of Cancer 2001;84(1) 100–105.

[101] Spitz MR, Bondy ML. The evolving discipline of molecular epidemiology of câncer. Carcinogenesis 2010;31(1) 127–134.

Chapter 2

The Crosstalk of c-MET with Related Receptor Tyrosine Kinases in Urothelial Bladder Cancer

Sheng-Hui Lan, Shan-Ying Wu, Giri Raghavaraju,
Nan-Haw Chow and Hsiao-Sheng Liu

Additional information is available at the end of the chapter

http://dx.doi.org/10.5772/53718

1. Introduction

RTKs are often deregulated in human malignancies, contributing to cancer development and progression. Deregulation of RTKs leads to aberrant receptor activity resulting in increased cell proliferation, inhibition of apoptosis, invasion, and enhanced tumor metastases. Because RTKs are membrane proteins, they represent attractive targets for cancer therapy, with a number of agents already approved for clinical use.

c-MET gene, located on chromosome 7q21-q31, encodes a single precursor protein and is post-transcriptionally digested and glycosylated. The mature receptor is composed of a 50 kDa extracellular α-chain and a transmembrane 140 kDa β-chain, which are linked by disulfide bonds [1]. The MET β-chain contains homologous domains that shared with other proteins, including a semaphorin (Sema) domain, a PSI domain (in plexins, semaphorins and integrins), four IPT repeats (in immunoglobulins, plexins and transcription factors), a transmembrane domain, a juxtamembrane domain, a tyrosine kinase domain and a carboxy-terminal tail region [2, 3].

The transforming property of c-MET was initially described in a human osteosarcoma cell line after chemically induced mutagenesis [4]. In this *in vitro* model, c-MET was found to be constitutively activated by translocation at (1;7), resulting in fused sequences of c-MET gene on chromosome 7q31 to the translocated promoter region on chromosome 1q25 [5]. Since then, support for c-MET signaling in human carcinogenesis comes from data of the cell culture [6], mice [7, 8], and sporadic and hereditary forms of renal carcinoma, where germline and somatic missense mutations were identified in c-MET's kinase domain [9, 10]. Furthermore, c-MET activity plays a significant role in promoting tumor invasion and metastasis

[11, 12]. In summary, c-MET regulates embryonic development and play important roles in the carcinogenesis, tumor progression, and a variety of cellular processes, including migration, proliferation, morphogenesis, and angiogenesis [13, 14].

HGF is predominantly secreted by mesenchymal cells, and c-MET is widely expressed on the surface of epithelial cancer cells [15]. Homodimerization of c-MET after binding to HGR leads to transphosphorylation of cytoplasmic tyrosine kinase domain at two specific sites (Y1234 and Y1235) and activation of down-stream signaling [16]. These events are essential during embryogenesis, and also play a critical role in normal tissue homeostasis of the hepatocytes, renal tubule cells, and myoblasts [17].

The phosphorylation of two tyrosine residues within COOH terminus (Y1349 and Y1356) is necessary and sufficient to mediate biological effects induced by of the c-MET activation [18]. These two residues recruit a number of adapter proteins, including Gab1, Grb2, Shc and the p85 subunit of phosphatidylinositol-3 kinase (PI3K) [17]. The involvement of diverse effectors allows the activation of different downstream pathways, including PI3K-Akt signaling, Ras-mitogen-activated protein kinase (MAPK) pathways, signal transducer and activator of transcription proteins (STATs) and the nuclear factor-kB (NF-kB) complex [17]. These signaling pathways are important during embryogenesis and in normal tissue homeostasis, such as cell proliferation, differentiation, transformation, migration and apoptosis.

Accumulating data have demonstrated that crosstalk between c-MET and other RTKs may contribute to tumor progression in some of human cancers [19-21]. As a result, evaluation of c-MET expression status and its crosstalk partners of RTKs may identify a subset of c-MET-positive cancer patients who may require co-targeting therapy.

2. Role of c-MET in human cancers

Overexpression of c-MET has been reported in different subtypes of lung cancer, including adenocarcinoma (67%), carcinoid (60%), large cell carcinoma (57%), squamous cell carcinoma (57%), and small cell lung cancer (SCLC) (25%) [22]. In terms of functional activity, positive staining could be demonstrated in the subtypes of adenocarcinoma (44%), large cell carcinoma (86%), squamous cell carcinoma (71%), carcinoid (40%), and SCLC (100%), respectively, using antibody for phospho-c-MET at the Y1003 (c-Cbl binding site). On the other hand, positive staining was observed in 33% of adenocarcinomas, 57% of large cell carcinoma and 50% of SCLCs using antibody for autophosphorylation of c-MET at the Y1230/1234/1235 site [22]. Importantly, missense germ-line mutations in the tyrosine kinase domain of c-MET have been described in patients with hereditary papillary renal carcinoma [9]; whereas sporadic mutations in the tyrosine kinase, juxtamembrane, or semaphorin domains of c-MET have been detected in gastric cancer, HCC and SCLCs [23-25]. Concerning biologic significance, activation of HGF/MET signalling pathway was shown to promote cell invasiveness *in vivo* and trigger tumor metastases through angiogenic pathways [26]. In addition, amplification of c-MET has been detected in the carcinomas of the stomach, esophagus, and colorectum, non–small-cell lung cancer, and glioblastoma, and is usually associated with acquired resistance to anticancer drugs-gefitinib or erlotinib [27-32].

Altered HGF secretion was reported in both solid and hematologic malignancies. Both tumor and mesenchymal cells are responsible for increased HGF production, leading to paracrine and/or autocrine activation of c-MET by HGF [33, 34, 35]. The enhanced c-MET signaling is tumorigenic and could induce tumor metastasis in athymic nude mice [11]. As a result, HGF and/or c-MET overexpression were suggested to be a prognostic biomarker for cancer patients [36-38], although not all studies got the same conclusion [39, 40].

3. Role of c-MET-related RTKs in cancer

In addition to c-MET, coexpression of c-MET and related RTKs was shown to have prognostic relevance in some human cancers [41-45]. For example, RON and MET were overexpressed in 55 % and 56 % of human ovarian cancer, respectively, and 42 % of them have coexpression of RON and MET ($P < 0.001$) [41]. Coexpression of RON/MET was associated with more aggressive phenotype of node-negative breast cancer patients. The 10-year disease-free survival in RON-/MET- breast cancer is significantly higher than that of RON+/MET+ group (79.3 % vs. 11.8 %) [42]. Furthermore, both MET and EGF family receptors are overexpressed in different human cancers. Coexpression of c-MET and HER2 were observed in breast cancer and cholangiocarcinoma, and is usually associated with poor prognosis [43]. Similarly, coexpression of c-MET and HER2 could be detected in gastric cancer, and activation of c-MET further increases the resistance to EGFR inhibitor-Lapatinib [44, 45].

4. Overexpression of c-MET as a prognostic indicator for urothelial carcinoma of the bladder

High levels of c-MET expression have been correlated with metastatic progression of tumors and poor survival in patients with carcinomas of the breast, extrahepatic biliary tract, stomach, endometrum, liver, colorectum, and kidney [46-53]. c-MET was also reported to play a positive role in the tumorigenesis of human bladder [54, 55]. For example, expression of c-met mRNA tended to positively correlate with differentiation of cancer cell lines in the absence of point mutation [55]. Expression of Met was positively associated with histologic grade, stage classification, tumor size, and nodular tumor growth ($P < 0.05$, respectively), and is an independent indicators for poor long-term survival ($P = 0.04$) [55]. Furthermore, pY1349 c-Met was found to be a prognostic marker in predicting metastasis-free and survival of bladder cancer in a large cohort study of 133 non-metastatic specimens of bladder cancer [56]. Taken together, c-met proto-oncogene plays an important role in the progression of bladder carcinogenesis. Evaluation of Met expression could identify a subset of bladder cancer patients who may require a more intensive treatment targeting strategy.

5. The signaling pathway of c-MET

5.1. c-MET-related signaling pathways

The signaling for growth depends on RAS-MAPK signaling pathway and plays an essential role in morphogenesis and epithelial-to-mesenchymal transition that results from loss of intracellular adhesion via cadherins, focal adhesion kinase, and integrins, in association with alteration of cell shape [57]. Activation of HGF/c-MET axis prevents cell apoptosis through PI3 kinase and subsequent Akt signaling events [58-60]. The crosstalk of c-MET and PI3K-Akt pathway with RAS-MAPK pathway has been implicated in patient survival [61, 62].

5.2. Crosstalk with other membrane proteins or receptor tyrosine kinases

c-MET is known to interact with other membrane proteins on the cell surface [63], including laminin receptor-$\alpha 6\beta 4$ integrin, semaphorin receptors of plexin B family, and v6 splice variant of hyaluronan receptor-CD44 [63, 64]. The crosstalk between c-MET and membrane proteins modulates the activation of both c-MET and its partners and allows for integration of signals present in the extracellular environment [65]. Crosstalk between c-MET and epidermal growth factor receptor (EGFR) has been implicated in several biological systems [66]. Furthermore, the crosstalk of c-MET with other RTKs regulates different physiological and/or pathological situations additively or synergistically. This interaction promotes trans-phosphorylation of kinase of each other by directly binding or transducing through their downstream signaling pathways indirectly. We review the potential role of c-MET and related RTKs, including RON, EGFR, Axl and platelet derived growth factor receptor-alpha (PDGFR-α), in urothelial carcinoma of the bladder, either independently or in combination in vivo (crosstalk) (Fig. 1).

6. RON

Recepteur d'Origine Nantais (RON) is a MET RTK subfamily member. Its ligand is macrophage-stimulating protein (MSP) which is expressed by renal tubular cells [67-69]. Activation of RON induces apoptotic resistance, superoxide anion production, and phagocytosis of macrophages through different molecules and related signaling pathways, *i.e.* Src, ERK, p38 and PI3K/AKT, which are related to tumorigenesis [70-72]. The crosstalk between c-MET and RON has been reported in different *in vitro* experimental models, and has been confirmed in the human cancers of the liver, ovary, breast and urinary bladder.

Heterodimerization plays a pivotal role in initiating the crosstalk and activation of related signal transduction pathways. Follenzi *et al.*, showed that activated c-MET directly cross-phosphorylates RON, and c-MET/RON heterodimmer activates the catalytic region of c-MET at Y1234/Y1235 and RON at Y1238/Y1239, respectively (Figure 1A). Moreover, both signal transducer docking sites of c-MET at Y1349/Y1356 and RON at Y1353/Y1360 are generated for downstream signaling molecules. Mutation of RON suppresses the transforming phenotype induced by c-MET [73]. In contrast, RON is specifically trans-phosphorylated by MET, but not by EGFR or HER2; and MET-specific kinase inhibitors also suppress the phosphorylation of RON [41]. In addition to HGF, other cytokines, including EGF, interleukin-1, interleukin-6 and tumor necrosis factor alpha (TNF- α), are able to induce the expression of both MET and RON in HCC, suggesting that MET and RON are regulated by similar cytokine networks [42].

Overexpression of RON increases the growth, motility and anti-apoptosis of cancer cells *in vitro* [74]. In primary human bladder cancer, overexpression of RON is detected in 32.8 % of the tumors, and 23.3 % of these positive tumors also showed high levels of MET expression as well. In addition, co-expressed RON and MET was significantly associated with decreased overall survival (P= 0.005) or metastasis-free survival (P = 0.01) [74]. Overexpression of RON and MET seems to be a universal event in uroepithelial cells [75]. These data support the potential significance of RON/MET crosstalk, and the occurrence as a biomarker in selection of appropriate treatment strategy for cancer patients.

7. EGFR

The EGFR (HER1 or ErbB-1 in humans) belongs to RTKs of ErbB family which consists of EGFR, HER2/c-neu (ErbB-2), Her3 (ErbB-3) and Her4 (ErbB-4) four subfamily members. EGF is the ligand of EGFR [76]. EGFR signaling pathway participates in the growth and progression of urothelial cancers. Mutations affecting EGFR expression or activity may initiate a cascade of events leading to autonomous cell proliferation, migration, invasion and apoptosis inhibition, leading to tumor progression [77, 78].

The crosstalk between EGFR and MET has been reported during development and tumorigenesis. Cooperative action of MET and EGFR controls the number of nephron (the functional unit of the kidney) and maintains the duct morphology during kidney development [79]. Three underlying mechanisms of crosstalk between MET and RTK have been reported: (1) Trans-phophorylation and activation: Both RON and EGFR can bind with MET, and form heterodimeric receptor complex to activate both tyrosine kinases through trans-phosphorylation. The crosstalk of EGFR or RON with c-MET was confirmed by co-immunoprecipitation assay (Figure 1A) [66, 80]; (2) c-MET activates EGFR through transcriptional activation of the ligand EGF: c-MET increases the production of EGF through Ras/Erk signaling-mediated promoter activation. EGF then is transported out of the cell to bind with EGFR in an autocrine or paracrine manner (Figure 1B) [81]; (3) EGFR activates c-MET through Ras/Erk MAPK signaling pathway to activate metalloproteinasea (TIMP)-3 which then cleavages the c-MET at ectodomain (Figure 1C). The truncated c-MET protein promotes the proliferation and cell transformation [82, 83].

Naik *et al.*, reported that positive staining for EGFR, HER2 and EGF could be detected in 23%, 60% and 47% of primary bladder cancer specimens, respectively [84]. The HER2/neu gene amplification and protein overexpression were demonstrated in high grade, invasive bladder cancer [85]. Overexpression of EGFR/ERBB2 correlates with higher tumor grading/

stage and poorer clinical outcome in bladder cancer patients [86, 87]. These evidences support the selection of EGFR as a molecular marker for diagnosis and/or prognosis of bladder carcinoma [88, 89]. Recently, EGFR inhibitor Iressa has shown a strong protective efficacy through cell cycle regulation in carcinogen induced rat bladder cancer model [90]. Therefore, EGFR, vascular endothelial growth factor (VEGF), mTOR and their-related signaling molecules are excellent therapeutic targets, in combination with cytotoxic chemotherapy, in the design of bladder cancer treatment [91]. Overexpression of RON and EGFR, as well as their crosstalk, has been reported in various human bladder cancer cell lines [74, 92]. It is noteworthy to clarify the potential of RTK co-targeting in the application of EGFR inhibitors in bladder cancer therapy.

8. AXL

AXL is a member of TAM RTK family, including AXL, Tyro3 and Merk. It has a unique structure of extracellular region that juxtaposes IgL and FNIII repeats [93, 94]. The protein S and Gas6 (growth-arrest-specific protein 6) are ligands for TAM receptor [95]. Gas6/AXL controls diverse cellular functions, including proliferation, survival, migration and anti-inflammation through different signaling pathways [96]. Gas6/AXL stimulates cell proliferation through MEK/Erk signaling pathway [97]. Gas6/AXL activates the PI3K/AKT and p38 signaling pathways to enhance the cell survival and migration, respectively [98, 99]. Gas6/AXL also suppresses Toll-like receptor and cytokine receptor signaling in innate immune cells through regulation of STAT1 [100, 101]. Overexpression of AXL has been reported in mesothelioma, NSCLC, breast carcinoma, and bladder cancer [20, 96, 102]. However, AXL can be activated by a ligand-independent manner when AXL interacts with adjacent cells in which AXL was overexpressed, suggesting that overexpression of AXL may be activated *per se* through auto-activation [103].

9. PDGFR-α

PDGF, a ligand of PDGFR-α and -β, results in auto-phosphorylation and signaling transduction of PDGFR [104]. PDGF/PDGFR signaling is involved in the development of various tissues, and is essential for epithelial-mesenchymal interaction during metamorphic skin remodeling, mesenchymal cell migration and proliferation [105]. In PDGF-α knock-out mice, neural tube and brain are abnormally accompanied by defect of the nervous system [106]. PDGF contributes to the development and progression of cancer by autocrine or paracrine signaling, and further promotes tumorigenesis through proliferation, angiogenesis and tumor stromal interaction [107].

In huamn uroepithelial cells, c-MET is frequently co-expressed with AXL, PDGFR-α, discoidin domain receptor tyrosine kinase 2 (DDR2), and/or insulin-like growth factor I receptor (IGF1R). Overexpression of AXL and PDGFR-α has been detected in various human cancers, and is associated with invasiveness and/or metastasis of carcinoma of the breast, kidney and bladder [20, 108, 109]. Overexpression of c-MET/PDGFR-α was demonstrated in all of 9 human bladder cancer cell lines tested [110]. We identified that both AXL and PDGFR may be c-MET related RTKs in a cDNA microarray analysis [20]. In sharp contrast to crosstalk between c-MET and RON or EGFR, both AXL and PDGFR do not directly bind with c-MET, and is transcriptionally activated by mitogen activated protein kinase/extracellular signal-regulated kinase (MEK/Erk) signaling pathway (Figure 1B) [20].

9.1. The relationship among environmental carcinogens, c-MET and RTKs

The environmental carcinogens, mainly from cigarette smoking, play important roles in the bladder cancer development, specifically urothelial carcinoma [111, 112]. Cigar smoking, pipe smoking, and secondhand smoke are implicated as risk factors for urothelial carcinoma. The incidence of urothelial cancer is approximately 4 times higher in smokers compared with non-smokers [113]. It is also reported that 50 % of all bladder cancers in men and 30 % in women are due to cigarette smoking [114]. All these evidences suggest that smoking is the most important risk factor for bladder cancer development. Genetic damage is the major cause of smoking-related cancer induction by which normal cellular pathways are altered to trigger cell growth and induce tumor formation [115]. In addition to bladder cancer, lung cancer formation is also induced by genetic modifications mostly caused by tobacco smoking [116]. Genetic mutations and amplifications in RTK related signaling, such as c-MET, EGFR, ErbB2, c-Kit, VEGFR, PI3K, and PTEN, contribute to lung cancer development by escaping from normal growth control and transforming into a malignant phenotype [117, 118]. Several autocrine loops, including stem cell factor (SCF)/c-Kit, IGF-I/IGF-IR, and HGF/c-MET, lead to the activation of PI3K/Akt signaling pathway and promote the cell growth, survival, and chemotherapy resistance in lung cancer. During lung cancer development, RTKs and their downstream effectors are selectively up-regulated. It is intriguing to clarify whether crosstalk of c-MET with RTKs in bladder cancer is also related to smoking. Altogether, it is noteworthy to clarify the relationship among smoking, c-MET, RTKs and bladder cancer development in the further study.

10. Conclusion and future direction

Overexpression of multiple RTKs has been reported in many human cancers, including bladder cancer. Cross-connection among individual signaling pathway activated by each RTK forms the signaling networks, which may complicate the development of anticancer strategies. With discussion above, more attention is focused to identify the prognostic targets and development of the targeted therapy for bladder cancer. In this review, we describe the current knowledge of interaction between c-MET and related RTKs. On the basis of complicated signaling network, the multimodal strategies should include systemic chemo- or biological therapies in combination with surgery and/or radiation applicable for invasive/metastatic bladder cancers [91]. Diverse therapeutic strategies have been developed to inhibit the HGF/c-MET signaling, including anti-HGF antibodies, HGF antagonists, anti-c-MET antibodies, and c-MET tyrosine kinase inhibitors. The c-MET pathway inhibitors have been reported to block the activities of other related tyrosine kinases. For example, MP470, a RAD51 inhibitor, suppresses the activity of c-MET and PDGFR [119]. MK-2461 suppresses the activity of both c-MET and RON [120]. BMS-777607 inhibits the activity of c-MET, RON and AXL [119, 121]. Furthermore, Foretinib, an oral multi-kinase inhibitor, inhibits the c-MET activity and its related RTKs (RON, EGFR, AXL and PDGFR) [122, 123]. Altogether, these inhibitors have potential to be used for bladder cancer therapy in the future. Cooperative action of c-MET with RON, EGFR, AXL and PDGFR-α has been reported to play important roles in bladder cancer progression, and thus deserves further investigation as the co-targeting therapy candidates. Understanding of the mechanisms underlying crosstalk of c-MET with RTKs is indispensible in the development of novel strategies against urothelial bladder cancer.

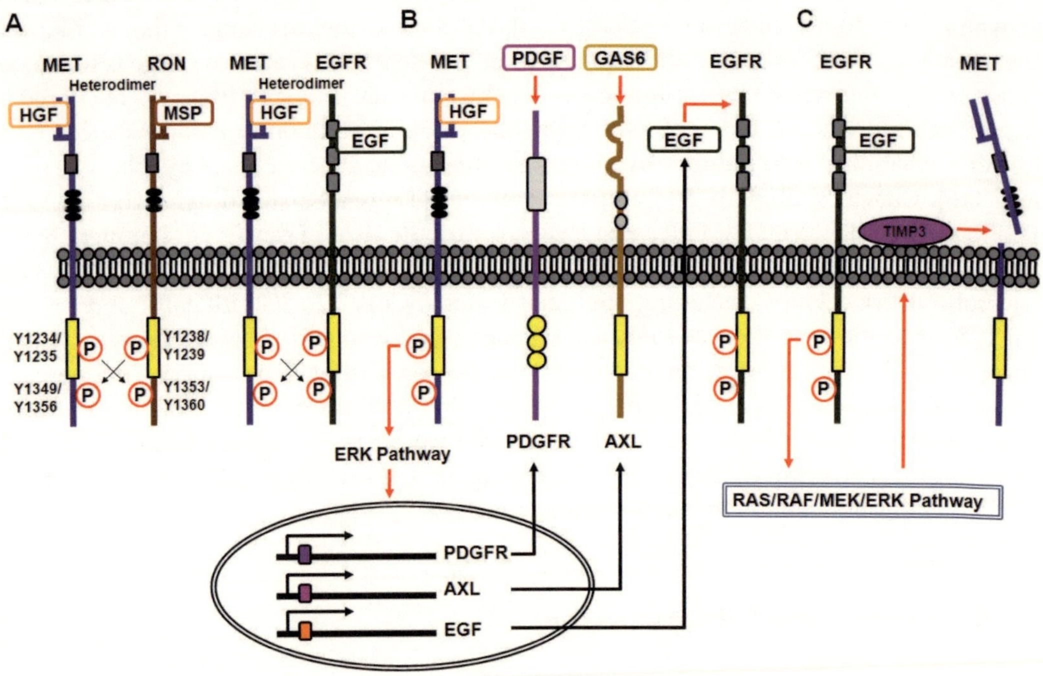

Figure 1. The crosstalk between c-MET and related receptor tyrosine kinases

A. Trans-phosphorylation by other RTKs. The ligands, such as HGF, MSP and EGF, activate the MET, RON and EGFR, respectively, through tyrosine phosphorylation. The activated receptors (MET, RON or EGFR) cross talk with other RTKs through trans-phosphorylation. B. Activation of other RTKs by c-MET through transcriptional regulation. HGF activates the c-MET and downstream Ras/Erk signaling pathway through tyrosine phosphorylation. Expression of PDGFR, AXL and EGF was enhanced through transcriptional regulation. Overexpression of PDGFR and AXL enhances their binding with cognate ligands (PDGF

http://dx.doi.org/10.5772/53718

and GAS6) and activation of their downstream signaling pathways. Overexpression of EGF further enhances the activity of EGFR in an autocrine or paracrine manner. C. Metalloproteinase cleavage regulates c-MET activation. EGF induces the phosphorylation of EGFR and activation of Ras/Erk signaling, and promotes the MET ectodomain shedding by cleavage of TIMP3 sensitive metalloproteinase.

Abbreviations

DDR2 (Discoidin domain receptor tyrosine kinase 2)

EGF (Epidermal growth factor)

EGFR (Epidermal growth factor receptor)

HCC (Hepatocellular carcinoma)

HGF (Hepatocyte growth factor)

HGFR (Hepatocyte growth factor receptor)

IGF1R (Insulin-like Growth Factor I Receptor)

IL-1 (Interleukin-1)

IL-6 (Interleukin-6)

MAPK (Mitogen-activated protein kinase)

MSP (Macrophage-stimulating protein)

NF-κB (Nuclear factor-κB)

PI3K (Phosphatidylinositol-3 kinase)

PDGFR (Platelet-derived growth factor receptor)

PTKs (Protein tyrosine kinases)

RON (Recepteur d'Origine Nantais)

RTKs (Receptor tyrosine kinases)

SCLCs (Small cell lung cancer cells)

STATs (Signal transducer and activator of transcription proteins)

TCC (Transitional cell carcinoma)

TIMPs (Tissue inhibitors of metalloproteinases)

TNF- α (Tumor necrosis factor alpha)

Acknowledgements

This review was supported by the grant from the National Science Council (NSC101-2320-B006-025-MY3)

Author details

Sheng-Hui Lan[1], Shan-Ying Wu[1], Giri Raghavaraju[2], Nan-Haw Chow[3] and Hsiao-Sheng Liu[1,2*]

*Address all correspondence to: a713@mail.ncku.edu.tw

1 Institute of Basic Medical sciences, College of Medicine, National Cheng Kung University, Tainan, Taiwan

2 Department of Microbiology and Immunology, College of Medicine, National Cheng Kung University, Tainan, Taiwan

3 Department of Pathology, College of medicine, National Cheng Kung University, Tainan, Taiwan

References

[1] Giordano, S., et al., Tyrosine kinase receptor indistinguishable from the c-met protein. Nature, 1989. 339(6220): p. 155-6.

[2] Maestrini, E., et al., A family of transmembrane proteins with homology to the MET-hepatocyte growth factor receptor. Proc Natl Acad Sci U S A, 1996. 93(2): p. 674-8.

[3] Sattler, M. and R. Salgia, c-Met and hepatocyte growth factor: potential as novel targets in cancer therapy. Curr Oncol Rep, 2007. 9(2): p. 102-8.

[4] Cooper, C.S., et al., Molecular cloning of a new transforming gene from a chemically transformed human cell line. Nature, 1984. 311(5981): p. 29-33.

[5] Park, M., et al., Sequence of MET protooncogene cDNA has features characteristic of the tyrosine kinase family of growth-factor receptors. Proc Natl Acad Sci U S A, 1987. 84(18): p. 6379-83.

[6] Maulik, G., et al., Role of the hepatocyte growth factor receptor, c-Met, in oncogenesis and potential for therapeutic inhibition. Cytokine Growth Factor Rev, 2002. 13(1): p. 41-59.

[7] Takayama, H., et al., Diverse tumorigenesis associated with aberrant development in mice overexpressing hepatocyte growth factor/scatter factor. Proc Natl Acad Sci U S A, 1997. 94(2): p. 701-6.

[8] Wang, R., et al., Activation of the Met receptor by cell attachment induces and sustains hepatocellular carcinomas in transgenic mice. J Cell Biol, 2001. 153(5): p. 1023-34.

[9] Schmidt, L., et al., Germline and somatic mutations in the tyrosine kinase domain of the MET proto-oncogene in papillary renal carcinomas. Nat Genet, 1997. 16(1): p. 68-73.

[10] Schmidt, L., et al., Two North American families with hereditary papillary renal carcinoma and identical novel mutations in the MET proto-oncogene. Cancer Res, 1998. 58(8): p. 1719-22.

[11] Rong, S., et al., Invasiveness and metastasis of NIH 3T3 cells induced by Met-hepatocyte growth factor/scatter factor autocrine stimulation. Proc Natl Acad Sci U S A, 1994. 91(11): p. 4731-5.

[12] Ma, P.C., et al., c-Met: structure, functions and potential for therapeutic inhibition. Cancer Metastasis Rev, 2003. 22(4): p. 309-25.

[13] Coyle, R.C., A. Latimer, and J.R. Jessen, Membrane-type 1 matrix metalloproteinase regulates cell migration during zebrafish gastrulation: evidence for an interaction with non-canonical Wnt signaling. Exp Cell Res, 2008. 314(10): p. 2150-62.

[14] Birchmeier, C., et al., Met, metastasis, motility and more. Nat Rev Mol Cell Biol, 2003. 4(12): p. 915-25.

[15] Prat, M., et al., The receptor encoded by the human c-MET oncogene is expressed in hepatocytes, epithelial cells and solid tumors. Int J Cancer, 1991. 49(3): p. 323-8.

[16] Longati, P., et al., Tyrosines1234-1235 are critical for activation of the tyrosine kinase encoded by the MET proto-oncogene (HGF receptor). Oncogene, 1994. 9(1): p. 49-57.

[17] Furge, K.A., Y.W. Zhang, and G.F. Vande Woude, Met receptor tyrosine kinase: enhanced signaling through adapter proteins. Oncogene, 2000. 19(49): p. 5582-9.

[18] Ponzetto, C., et al., A multifunctional docking site mediates signaling and transformation by the hepatocyte growth factor/scatter factor receptor family. Cell, 1994. 77(2): p. 261-71.

[19] Jung, K.H., B.H. Park, and S.S. Hong, Progress in cancer therapy targeting c-Met signaling pathway. Arch Pharm Res, 2012. 35(4): p. 595-604.

[20] Yeh, C.Y., et al., Transcriptional activation of the Axl and PDGFR-alpha by c-Met through a ras- and Src-independent mechanism in human bladder cancer. BMC Cancer, 2011. 11: p. 139.

[21] Tanizaki, J., et al., Differential roles of trans-phosphorylated EGFR, HER2, HER3, and RET as heterodimerisation partners of MET in lung cancer with MET amplification. Br J Cancer, 2011. 105(6): p. 807-13.

[22] Ma, P.C., et al., Functional expression and mutations of c-Met and its therapeutic inhibition with SU11274 and small interfering RNA in non-small cell lung cancer. Cancer Res, 2005. 65(4): p. 1479-88.

[23] Lee, J.H., et al., A novel germ line juxtamembrane Met mutation in human gastric cancer. Oncogene, 2000. 19(43): p. 4947-53.

[24] Park, W.S., et al., Somatic mutations in the kinase domain of the Met/hepatocyte growth factor receptor gene in childhood hepatocellular carcinomas. Cancer Res, 1999. 59(2): p. 307-10.

[25] Ma, P.C., et al., c-MET mutational analysis in small cell lung cancer: novel juxtamembrane domain mutations regulating cytoskeletal functions. Cancer Res, 2003. 63(19): p. 6272-81.

[26] Zhang, Y.W., et al., Hepatocyte growth factor/scatter factor mediates angiogenesis through positive VEGF and negative thrombospondin 1 regulation. Proc Natl Acad Sci U S A, 2003. 100(22): p. 12718-23.

[27] Smolen, G.A., et al., Amplification of MET may identify a subset of cancers with extreme sensitivity to the selective tyrosine kinase inhibitor PHA-665752. Proc Natl Acad Sci U S A, 2006. 103(7): p. 2316-21.

[28] Miller, C.T., et al., Genomic amplification of MET with boundaries within fragile site FRA7G and upregulation of MET pathways in esophageal adenocarcinoma. Oncogene, 2006. 25(3): p. 409-18.

[29] Umeki, K., G. Shiota, and H. Kawasaki, Clinical significance of c-met oncogene alterations in human colorectal cancer. Oncology, 1999. 56(4): p. 314-21.

[30] Beroukhim, R., et al., Assessing the significance of chromosomal aberrations in cancer: methodology and application to glioma. Proc Natl Acad Sci U S A, 2007. 104(50): p. 20007-12.

[31] Engelman, J.A., et al., MET amplification leads to gefitinib resistance in lung cancer by activating ERBB3 signaling. Science, 2007. 316(5827): p. 1039-43.

[32] Bean, J., et al., MET amplification occurs with or without T790M mutations in EGFR mutant lung tumors with acquired resistance to gefitinib or erlotinib. Proc Natl Acad Sci U S A, 2007. 104(52): p. 20932-7.

[33] Ferracini, R., et al., The Met/HGF receptor is over-expressed in human osteosarcomas and is activated by either a paracrine or an autocrine circuit. Oncogene, 1995. 10(4): p. 739-49.

[34] Furge, K.A., et al., Suppression of Ras-mediated tumorigenicity and metastasis through inhibition of the Met receptor tyrosine kinase. Proc Natl Acad Sci U S A, 2001. 98(19): p. 10722-7.

[35] Moghul, A., et al., Modulation of c-MET proto-oncogene (HGF receptor) mRNA abundance by cytokines and hormones: evidence for rapid decay of the 8 kb c-MET transcript. Oncogene, 1994. 9(7): p. 2045-52.

[36] Shattuck, D.L., et al., Met receptor contributes to trastuzumab resistance of Her2-overexpressing breast cancer cells. Cancer Res, 2008. 68(5): p. 1471-7.

[37] Siegfried, J.M., et al., Association of immunoreactive hepatocyte growth factor with poor survival in resectable non-small cell lung cancer. Cancer Res, 1997. 57(3): p. 433-9.

[38] Sawada, K., et al., c-Met overexpression is a prognostic factor in ovarian cancer and an effective target for inhibition of peritoneal dissemination and invasion. Cancer Res, 2007. 67(4): p. 1670-9.

[39] Nakamura, Y., et al., c-Met activation in lung adenocarcinoma tissues: an immunohistochemical analysis. Cancer Sci, 2007. 98(7): p. 1006-13.

[40] Resnick, M.B., et al., Epidermal growth factor receptor, c-MET, beta-catenin, and p53 expression as prognostic indicators in stage II colon cancer: a tissue microarray study. Clin Cancer Res, 2004. 10(9): p. 3069-75.

[41] Maggiora, P., et al., The RON and MET oncogenes are co-expressed in human ovarian carcinomas and cooperate in activating invasiveness. Exp Cell Res, 2003. 288(2): p. 382-9.

[42] Lee, W.Y., et al., Prognostic significance of co-expression of RON and MET receptors in node-negative breast cancer patients. Clin Cancer Res, 2005. 11(6): p. 2222-8.

[43] Lengyel, E., et al., C-Met overexpression in node-positive breast cancer identifies patients with poor clinical outcome independent of Her2/neu. Int J Cancer, 2005. 113(4): p. 678-82.

[44] Chen, C.T., et al., MET Activation Mediates Resistance to Lapatinib Inhibition of HER2-Amplified Gastric Cancer Cells. Mol Cancer Ther, 2012. 11(3): p. 660-9.

[45] Carneiro, F. and M. Sobrinho-Simoes, The prognostic significance of amplification and overexpression of c-met and c-erb B-2 in human gastric carcinomas. Cancer, 2000. 88(1): p. 238-40.

[46] Ghoussoub, R.A., et al., Expression of c-met is a strong independent prognostic factor in breast carcinoma. Cancer, 1998. 82(8): p. 1513-20.

[47] Hida, Y., et al., Clinical significance of hepatocyte growth factor and c-Met expression in extrahepatic biliary tract cancers. Oncol Rep, 1999. 6(5): p. 1051-6.

[48] Nakajima, M., et al., The prognostic significance of amplification and overexpression of c-met and c-erb B-2 in human gastric carcinomas. Cancer, 1999. 85(9): p. 1894-902.

[49] Taniguchi, K., et al., The relation between the growth patterns of gastric carcinoma and the expression of hepatocyte growth factor receptor (c-met), autocrine motility factor receptor, and urokinase-type plasminogen activator receptor. Cancer, 1998. 82(11): p. 2112-22.

[50] Wagatsuma, S., et al., Tumor angiogenesis, hepatocyte growth factor, and c-Met expression in endometrial carcinoma. Cancer, 1998. 82(3): p. 520-30.

[51] Ueki, T., et al., Expression of hepatocyte growth factor and its receptor c-met protooncogene in hepatocellular carcinoma. Hepatology, 1997. 25(4): p. 862-6.

[52] Di Renzo, M.F., et al., Overexpression and amplification of the met/HGF receptor gene during the progression of colorectal cancer. Clin Cancer Res, 1995. 1(2): p. 147-54.

[53] Natali, P.G., et al., Overexpression of the met/HGF receptor in renal cell carcinomas. Int J Cancer, 1996. 69(3): p. 212-7.

[54] Joseph, A., et al., Expression of scatter factor in human bladder carcinoma. J Natl Cancer Inst, 1995. 87(5): p. 372-7.

[55] Cheng, H.L., et al., Overexpression of c-met as a prognostic indicator for transitional cell carcinoma of the urinary bladder. A comparison with p53 nuclear accumulation. J Clin Oncol, 2002, 20(60): p. 1544-50.

[56] Miyata, Y., et al., Phosphorylated hepatocyte growth factor receptor/c-Met is associated with tumor growth and prognosis in patients with bladder cancer: correlation with matrix metalloproteinase-2 and -7 and E-cadherin. Hum Pathol, 2009. 40(4): p. 496-504.

[57] Boccaccio, C. and P.M. Comoglio, Invasive growth: a MET-driven genetic programme for cancer and stem cells. Nat Rev Cancer, 2006. 6(8): p. 637-45.

[58] Fan, S., et al., The cytokine hepatocyte growth factor/scatter factor inhibits apoptosis and enhances DNA repair by a common mechanism involving signaling through phosphatidyl inositol 3' kinase. Oncogene, 2000. 19(18): p. 2212-23.

[59] Derksen, P.W., et al., The hepatocyte growth factor/Met pathway controls proliferation and apoptosis in multiple myeloma. Leukemia, 2003. 17(4): p. 764-74.

[60] Xiao, G.H., et al., Anti-apoptotic signaling by hepatocyte growth factor/Met via the phosphatidylinositol 3-kinase/Akt and mitogen-activated protein kinase pathways. Proc Natl Acad Sci U S A, 2001. 98(1): p. 247-52.

[61] Zeng, Q., et al., Hepatocyte growth factor inhibits anoikis in head and neck squamous cell carcinoma cells by activation of ERK and Akt signaling independent of NFkappa B. J Biol Chem, 2002. 277(28): p. 25203-8.

[62] Tulasne, D. and B. Foveau, The shadow of death on the MET tyrosine kinase receptor. Cell Death Differ, 2008. 15(3): p. 427-34.

[63] Knudsen, B.S. and G. Vande Woude, Showering c-MET-dependent cancers with drugs. Curr Opin Genet Dev, 2008. 18(1): p. 87-96.

[64] Comoglio, P.M., S. Giordano, and L. Trusolino, Drug development of MET inhibitors: targeting oncogene addiction and expedience. Nat Rev Drug Discov, 2008. 7(6): p. 504-16.

[65] Migliore, C. and S. Giordano, Molecular cancer therapy: can our expectation be MET? Eur J Cancer, 2008. 44(5): p. 641-51.

[66] Guo, A., et al., Signaling networks assembled by oncogenic EGFR and c-Met. Proc Natl Acad Sci U S A, 2008. 105(2): p. 692-7.

[67] Ronsin, C., et al., A novel putative receptor protein tyrosine kinase of the met family. Oncogene, 1993. 8(5): p. 1195-202.

[68] Wang, M.H., et al., Identification of the ron gene product as the receptor for the human macrophage stimulating protein. Science, 1994. 266(5182): p. 117-9.

[69] Rampino, T., et al., Macrophage-stimulating protein is produced by tubular cells and activates mesangial cells. J Am Soc Nephrol, 2002. 13(3): p. 649-57.

[70] Brunelleschi, S., et al., Macrophage stimulating protein (MSP) evokes superoxide anion production by human macrophages of different origin. Br J Pharmacol, 2001. 134(6): p. 1285-95.

[71] Chen, Y.Q., J.H. Fisher, and M.H. Wang, Activation of the RON receptor tyrosine kinase inhibits inducible nitric oxide synthase (iNOS) expression by murine peritoneal exudate macrophages: phosphatidylinositol-3 kinase is required for RON-mediated inhibition of iNOS expression. J Immunol, 1998. 161(9): p. 4950-9.

[72] Lutz, M.A. and P.H. Correll, Activation of CR3-mediated phagocytosis by MSP requires the RON receptor, tyrosine kinase activity, phosphatidylinositol 3-kinase, and protein kinase C zeta. J Leukoc Biol, 2003. 73(6): p. 802-14.

[73] Follenzi, A., et al., Cross-talk between the proto-oncogenes Met and Ron. Oncogene, 2000. 19(27): p. 3041-9.

[74] Cheng, H.L., et al., Co-expression of RON and MET is a prognostic indicator for patients with transitional-cell carcinoma of the bladder. Br J Cancer, 2005. 92(10): p. 1906-14.

[75] Comperat, E., et al., Prognostic value of MET, RON and histoprognostic factors for urothelial carcinoma in the upper urinary tract. J Urol, 2008. 179(3): p. 868-72; discussion 872.

[76] Herbst, R.S., Review of epidermal growth factor receptor biology. Int J Radiat Oncol Biol Phys, 2004. 59(2 Suppl): p. 21-6.

[77] Mendelsohn, J., The epidermal growth factor receptor as a target for cancer therapy. Endocr Relat Cancer, 2001. 8(1): p. 3-9.

[78] Kulik, G., A. Klippel, and M.J. Weber, Antiapoptotic signalling by the insulin-like growth factor I receptor, phosphatidylinositol 3-kinase, and Akt. Mol Cell Biol, 1997. 17(3): p. 1595-606.

[79] Ishibe, S., et al., Met and the epidermal growth factor receptor act cooperatively to regulate final nephron number and maintain collecting duct morphology. Development, 2009. 136(2): p. 337-45.

[80] Jo, M., et al., Cross-talk between epidermal growth factor receptor and c-Met signal pathways in transformed cells. J Biol Chem, 2000. 275(12): p. 8806-11.

[81] Reznik, T.E., et al., Transcription-dependent epidermal growth factor receptor activation by hepatocyte growth factor. Mol Cancer Res, 2008. 6(1): p. 139-50.

[82] Nath, D., et al., Shedding of c-Met is regulated by crosstalk between a G-protein coupled receptor and the EGF receptor and is mediated by a TIMP-3 sensitive metalloproteinase. J Cell Sci, 2001. 114(Pt 6): p. 1213-20.

[83] Merlin, S., et al., Deletion of the ectodomain unleashes the transforming, invasive, and tumorigenic potential of the MET oncogene. Cancer Sci, 2009. 100(4): p. 633-8.

[84] Naik, D.S., et al., Epidermal growth factor receptor expression in urinary bladder cancer. Indian J Urol, 2011. 27(2): p. 208-14.

[85] Latif, Z., et al., HER2/neu gene amplification and protein overexpression in G3 pT2 transitional cell carcinoma of the bladder: a role for anti-HER2 therapy? Eur J Cancer, 2004. 40(1): p. 56-63.

[86] Zheng, Y., et al., Dihydrotestosterone upregulates the expression of epidermal growth factor receptor and ERBB2 in androgen receptor-positive bladder cancer cells. Endocr Relat Cancer, 2011. 18(4): p. 451-64.

[87] Jimenez, R.E., et al., Her-2/neu overexpression in muscle-invasive urothelial carcinoma of the bladder: prognostic significance and comparative analysis in primary and metastatic tumors. Clin Cancer Res, 2001. 7(8): p. 2440-7.

[88] Neal, D.E. and K. Mellon, Epidermal growth factor receptor and bladder cancer: a review. Urol Int, 1992. 48(4): p. 365-71.

[89] Kassouf, W., et al., Distinctive expression pattern of ErbB family receptors signifies an aggressive variant of bladder cancer. J Urol, 2008. 179(1): p. 353-8.

[90] Lu, Y., et al., Modulation of gene expression and cell-cycle signaling pathways by the EGFR inhibitor gefitinib (Iressa) in rat urinary bladder cancer. Cancer Prev Res (Phila), 2012. 5(2): p. 248-59.

[91] Vishnu, P., J. Mathew, and W.W. Tan, Current therapeutic strategies for invasive and metastatic bladder cancer. Onco Targets Ther, 2011. 4: p. 97-113.

[92] Hsu, P.Y., et al., Collaboration of RON and epidermal growth factor receptor in human bladder carcinogenesis. J Urol, 2006. 176(5): p. 2262-7.

[93] O'Bryan, J.P., et al., axl, a transforming gene isolated from primary human myeloid leukemia cells, encodes a novel receptor tyrosine kinase. Mol Cell Biol, 1991. 11(10): p. 5016-31.

[94] Hafizi, S., et al., Interaction of Axl receptor tyrosine kinase with C1-TEN, a novel C1 domain-containing protein with homology to tensin. Biochem Biophys Res Commun, 2002. 299(5): p. 793-800.

[95] Faust, M., et al., The murine ufo receptor: molecular cloning, chromosomal localization and in situ expression analysis. Oncogene, 1992. 7(7): p. 1287-93.

[96] Linger, R.M., et al., Taking aim at Mer and Axl receptor tyrosine kinases as novel therapeutic targets in solid tumors. Expert Opin Ther Targets, 2010. 14(10): p. 1073-90.

[97] Fridell, Y.W., et al., Differential activation of the Ras/extracellular-signal-regulated protein kinase pathway is responsible for the biological consequences induced by the Axl receptor tyrosine kinase. Mol Cell Biol, 1996. 16(1): p. 135-45.

[98] Berclaz, G., et al., Estrogen dependent expression of the receptor tyrosine kinase axl in normal and malignant human breast. Ann Oncol, 2001. 12(6): p. 819-24.

[99] Allen, M.P., et al., Novel mechanism for gonadotropin-releasing hormone neuronal migration involving Gas6/Ark signaling to p38 mitogen-activated protein kinase. Mol Cell Biol, 2002. 22(2): p. 599-613.

[100] Sharif, M.N., et al., Twist mediates suppression of inflammation by type I IFNs and Axl. J Exp Med, 2006. 203(8): p. 1891-901.

[101] Rothlin, C.V., et al., TAM receptors are pleiotropic inhibitors of the innate immune response. Cell, 2007. 131(6): p. 1124-36.

[102] Ou, W.B., et al., AXL regulates mesothelioma proliferation and invasiveness. Oncogene, 2011. 30(14): p. 1643-52.

[103] Bellosta, P., et al., The receptor tyrosine kinase ARK mediates cell aggregation by homophilic binding. Mol Cell Biol, 1995. 15(2): p. 614-25.

[104] Farooqi, A.A., et al., PDGF: the nuts and bolts of signalling toolbox. Tumour Biol, 2011. 32(6): p. 1057-70.

[105] Utoh, R., et al., Platelet-derived growth factor signaling as a cue of the epithelial-mesenchymal interaction required for anuran skin metamorphosis. Dev Dyn, 2003. 227(2): p. 157-69.

[106] Fruttiger, M., et al., Defective oligodendrocyte development and severe hypomyelination in PDGF-A knockout mice. Development, 1999. 126(3): p. 457-67.

[107] Yu, J., C. Ustach, and H.R. Kim, Platelet-derived growth factor signaling and human cancer. J Biochem Mol Biol, 2003. 36(1): p. 49-59.

[108] Meric, F., et al., Expression profile of tyrosine kinases in breast cancer. Clin Cancer Res, 2002. 8(2): p. 361-7.

[109] Chung, B.I., et al., Expression of the proto-oncogene Axl in renal cell carcinoma. DNA Cell Biol, 2003. 22(8): p. 533-40.

[110] Black, P.C., et al., Sensitivity to epidermal growth factor receptor inhibitor requires E-cadherin expression in urothelial carcinoma cells. Clin Cancer Res, 2008. 14(5): p. 1478-86.

[111] Kiriluk, K.J., et al., Bladder cancer risk from occupational and environmental exposures. Urol Oncol, 2012. 30(2): p. 199-211.

[112] Wilhelm-Benartzi, C.S., et al., Association of secondhand smoke exposures with DNA methylation in bladder carcinomas. Cancer Causes Control, 2011. 22(8): p. 1205-13.

[113] Burch, J.D., et al., Risk of bladder cancer by source and type of tobacco exposure: a case-control study. Int J Cancer, 1989. 44(4): p. 622-8.

[114] Zeegers, M.P., et al., The impact of characteristics of cigarette smoking on urinary tract cancer risk: a meta-analysis of epidemiologic studies. Cancer, 2000. 89(3): p. 630-9.

[115] Alberg, A.J. and J.R. Hebert, Cigarette smoking and bladder cancer: a new twist in an old saga? J Natl Cancer Inst, 2009. 101(22): p. 1525-6.

[116] Wojtalla, A. and A. Arcaro, Targeting phosphoinositide 3-kinase signalling in lung cancer. Crit Rev Oncol Hematol, 2011. 80(2): p. 278-90.

[117] Hodkinson, P.S., A. Mackinnon, and T. Sethi, Targeting growth factors in lung cancer. Chest, 2008. 133(5): p. 1209-16.

[118] Pisick, E., S. Jagadeesh, and R. Salgia, Receptor tyrosine kinases and inhibitors in lung cancer. ScientificWorldJournal, 2004. 4: p. 589-604.

[119] Liu, X., R.C. Newton, and P.A. Scherle, Development of c-MET pathway inhibitors. Expert Opin Investig Drugs, 2011. 20(9): p. 1225-41.

[120] Pan, B.S., et al., MK-2461, a novel multitargeted kinase inhibitor, preferentially inhibits the activated c-Met receptor. Cancer Res, 2010. 70(4): p. 1524-33.

[121] Schroeder, G.M., et al., Discovery of N-(4-(2-amino-3-chloropyridin-4-yloxy)-3-fluorophenyl)-4-ethoxy-1-(4-fluorophenyl)-2-oxo-1,2-dihydropyridine-3-carboxamide (BMS-777607), a selective and orally efficacious inhibitor of the Met kinase superfamily. J Med Chem, 2009. 52(5): p. 1251-4.

[122] Qian, F., et al., Inhibition of tumor cell growth, invasion, and metastasis by EXEL-2880 (XL880, GSK1363089), a novel inhibitor of HGF and VEGF receptor tyrosine kinases. Cancer Res, 2009. 69(20): p. 8009-16.

[123] Zillhardt, M., et al., Foretinib (GSK1363089), an orally available multikinase inhibitor of c-Met and VEGFR-2, blocks proliferation, induces anoikis, and impairs ovarian cancer metastasis. Clin Cancer Res, 2011. 17(12): p. 4042-51.

Chapter 3

Loss of Imprinting as an Epigenetic Marker in Bladder Cancer

Mariana Bisarro dos Reis and
Cláudia Aparecida Rainho

Additional information is available at the end of the chapter

http://dx.doi.org/10.5772/55814

1. Introduction

Currently, it is well recognized that epigenetic changes and genetic alterations are involved in the initiation and progression of human cancer. Epigenetics refers to the study of changes in gene expression caused by mechanisms other than classical mutations in the DNA sequence; these changes are potentially reversible but are generally stably maintained during cell division. The most common biological processes resulting from epigenetic mechanisms include X-chromosome inactivation, cellular differentiation, maintenance of cell identity and genomic imprinting.

Genomic imprinting is an epigenetic process of gene regulation in which the parental origin of an allele determines whether the allele will be expressed or repressed [1]. The imprinting is maintained by epigenetic modifications such as DNA methylation and repressive histone marks that are transmitted to the gametes from the parental germ lines to ensure the expression of a gene in a parent-specific manner. In somatic cells, the imprinted pattern is inherited during mitotic division leading to the specific-monoallelic expression of the opposite allele on the homologous chromosome [2]. However, in adult tissues, the patterns of imprinting of a gene may be complex, in which the specific-monoallelic expression is restricted to a limited number of cell types while biallelic transcripts produced from different promoters can be observed in other cells or tissues [3]. Furthermore, the majority of the genes regulated by imprinting are clustered with a long non-coding RNA; the expression of the genes in these clusters is controlled *in cis* by an imprinting control region (ICR) containing a differentially methylated region (DMR) that exhibits parent-specific DNA methylation. Thus, epigenetic modifications lead to the expression from only one of the two chromosome homologues depending on whether they are the maternally or paternally inherited copy of the gene.

In humans, the appropriate expression of imprinted genes is important for normal development. The loss of genomic imprinting exposes the organism to a greater risk of diseases because the disruption of normal patterns could lead to gain or loss of expression of the alleles and subsequently to imbalances in the amount of the gene product. There are numerous diseases associated with defects of imprinted genes including growth and metabolism disorders; various childhood and adult cancers; and disorders in neurodevelopment, cognition, and behavior as well as certain major psychiatric disorders.

Currently, approximately 80 imprinted genes have been characterized in the mouse genome. Two-thirds of them show conserved imprinting patterns between mice and humans, whereas others show imprinting patterns specific to humans. A large number of genes are also predicted to be imprinted [4].

This chapter will describe the molecular basis of genomic imprinting including epigenetic marks associated with the silencing of imprinted genes, the loss of imprinting as a potential marker of risk and prognostic biomarkers in human cancer with a focus on bladder cancer.

2. Imprinted genes: regulation and function

Genomic imprinting has four important principles. First, it must be able to influence gene expression. Second, it must be heritable in somatic lineages such that the memory of the parental origin is propagated into daughter cells. Third, it should be initiated on the paternally and maternally inherited chromosomes during gametogenesis or immediately after fertilization. Finally, imprinting must be erased in the germ line so that parental identity can be established in the gametes for the next generation [5].

Mechanisms responsible for establishing and maintaining imprinting include DNA methylation, chromatin modifications, insulation and the expression of non-coding RNAs (ncRNAs). DNA methylation is a reversible reaction that is catalyzed by DNA methyltransferases, an enzyme family that adds a methyl group to the 5-carbon of a cytosine that is immediately followed by a guanine. In the human cells, the methylation is almost restricted to these CpG dinucleotides, which are largely under-represented in the genome except at genomic regions called CpG islands, some of them associated with gene promoters [6]. In 2004, Kaneda *et al.* [7] demonstrated that a specific DNA methyltransferase, Dnmt3a, is essential for the establishment of both maternal and paternal imprinting. Once imprinting is established in the germ line, it is necessary to maintain the marks after reprogramming and *de novo* methylation that occurs after the pre-implantation of the embryo [8]. In somatic cells, imprinting is maintained and modified during development [9], and tissue-specific imprinting is frequently observed [10].

Although DNA methylation is the most important mechanism for imprinting, it does not appear to be the only mechanism. DMRs are often, but not exclusively, associated with chromatin modifications [11]. The majority of imprinted genes are clustered into megabase-long regions in the genome, which are essential to coordinate their regulation [12]. According to Barlow [2], more than 80% of the known imprinted genes are clustered into 16 genomic regions that contain two or more genes. The cluster organization reflects the coordinated regulation of the genes in a chromosomal domain [9]. These clusters share a number of features, including a ncRNA that is expressed from the parental allele opposite the protein-coding genes and the ICR [13]. The ICRs exhibit parental-specific epigenetic modifications (DNA methylation and histone modifications) that govern their activity [14].

Chromatin is mainly composed of histone proteins (H2A, H2B, H3, and H4) that are subjected to a variety of post-translational modifications on specific amino acid residues that are located in the histone tails (NH2 terminal regions). These modifications include acetylation, methylation, phosphorylation, sumoylation, ubiquitination and ADP ribosylation [15,16]. In somatic cells, the germline DMRs are marked by allele-specific histone modifications. In both maternal and paternal germ line DMRs, the unmethylated allele is associated with hallmarks of permissive chromatin, such as dimethylation of lysine 4 of histone H3 (H3K4me2) and H3/H4 acetylation [17]. Still, allele-specific DNA methylation at the ICRs in mice is associated with histone H4-lysine-20 and H3-lysine-9 trimethylation [18]. These marks, which also include histone H3-lysine-27 trimethylation (H3K27me3), histone H4-lysine-20 trimethylation (H4K20me3) and histone H3-lysine-9 di/trimethylation (H3K9me2/me3), are frequently associated with heterochromatic regions and a repressed status [19].

In a study conducted by Henckel *et al.* [20] with mid-gestation embryos obtained from Dnmt3L -/- females (DNA methylation at ICRs is not established during oogenesis), they observed a lack of repressive histone modifications suggesting that there is a mechanistic link between DNA and histone methylation at ICRs. It has been suggested that the methylation of the CpG dinucleotides in these control regions can affect the expression of the gene by preventing the binding of insulator proteins to differentially methylated regions. This methylation event precludes the binding of transcription factors to the promoter and changes the chromatin structure by recruiting methyl-CpG binding domain (MBD) proteins that bind to methylated CpGs and recruit other proteins [1]. Thus, the regulation of expression could depend on the local concentration of CpGs within the DMR.

The clusters are regulated by two main imprinting mechanisms. First, imprinting marks in the DMR can act as insulator elements and regulate the expression of imprinted genes, and second, the DMR can serve as a promoter for regulatory non-coding RNAs (ncRNAs). In the first model, the imprinted genes share regulatory elements, and the insulator controls access to these elements.

The *H19/IGF2* locus is the well-documented example of this model. Located at 11p15.5 in the human genome, these genes are connected and are expressed in a mutually exclusive manner [21]. In humans and rats, the transcription of *IFG2* and *H19* genes are coordinated by a group of enhancers located downstream to *H19* and a DMR located upstream to this gene [22]. The enhancers, lying between +7 and +9.5 kb from the promoter, include those sites that control expression in endodermal [23] and mesodermal [24] tissues. The second important element in this insulator model is the ICR or DMR. This element resides at -2 Kb to -4 Kb from the *H19* transcriptional start site and is crucial for establishing the molecular imprint of the *H19* gene in the early embryo [25]. This region was shown to block enhancer activity for the *H19* and

IFG2 genes and contains seven CTCF-binding sites that are required for this activity. When these CTCF-binding sites are methylated, they no longer bind the CTCF insulator protein [26]. CTCF is a ubiquitous, highly conserved transcription factor that plays multiple roles in gene regulation, such as in activation, repression, silencing, chromatin insulation, and long-range chromosome interactions [27]. On the maternal allele, the presence of CTCF blocks the enhancer from interacting with *IFG2* promoters and silences gene expression [28]. In contrast, CTCF does not bind to the methylated, paternally inherited chromosome. As a result, the enhancers are free to interact with the *IFG2* promoter, and the *H19* promoter is repressed [5]. The three-dimensional arrangement of the chromatin fiber created by CTCF-mediated interactions also plays an important role in imprinted gene expression at the *H19/IFG2* locus [29]. In 2004, by using the chromosome conformation capture (3C) method in a mouse model, it was demonstrated that the *Igf2* DMR1 (one of the three DMRs found in mouse, located upstream to the promoter 1 of the *Igf2* gene) is able to interact with the *H19*-DMR [30]. Another study also suggested that chromosomal looping is involved in the imprinting mechanism and that the CTCF sites can mediate allele-specific chromosome interactions that control the accessibility of the *IFG2* promoter to the shared enhancer [31,32].

The second mechanism regulating the expression of imprinted gene clusters involves a ncRNA. These ncRNAs function to silence large domains of the genome through their interaction with chromatin [33]. At present, several classes of ncRNAs have been identified within imprinted regions, including small nucleolar RNAs (snoRNAs), microRNAs (miRNAs), small interfering RNAs (siRNAs), Piwi-interacting RNAs (piRNAs), antisense ncRNAs and long non-coding RNAs (lncRNAs). While the expression of some plays a functional role in the regulation of genomic imprinting, the function of others remains to be determined [34]. It has been demonstrated that each imprinted cluster expresses at least on ncRNA that display reciprocally imprinted expression patterns relative to the neighboring protein-coding genes and that some of these genes are transcribed in an antisense orientation relative to the protein-coding gene [35]. The most studied and well-understood clusters in this class are the *Ifg2r* and *Kcnq1* clusters. *Ifg*2r and two neighboring genes, *Slc22a2* and *Slc22a3* (solute carrier 22a2 and 22a3), are maternally expressed. This region also harbors one paternally expressed transcript, *Air* (antisense to *Ifg2r* RNA) [36]. *Air* localizes to the silenced *Slc22a3* promoter, recruits the KMT1C lysine methyltransferase and leads to targeted H3K9 methylation and allele-specific gene silencing by chromatin remodeling [37]. Similar to the *Air–Ifg2r* locus, the *Kcnq1* locus contains a series of maternally expressed genes (at least eight) and a unique non-coding paternally expressed gene, *Kcnq1ot1* [34]. This locus is governed by the maternally methylated ICR, KvDMR1, located within an intron of the *Kcnq1* gene. The promoter for the *Kcnq1ot1* gene resides within KvDMR1[14]. According [38], *Kcnq1ot1* is required for epigenetic silencing of neighboring genes upstream and downstream of the *Kcnq1* locus.

The imprinted genes showed that complex regulation and functional consequences are associated with imprinting-induced changes in the expression level. One consequence of genomic imprinting is that viable embryos must receive two haploid genome complements that come from parents of the opposite sex [39]. Generally, the imprinted genes are highly expressed during embryonic development and are down-regulated after birth.

http://dx.doi.org/10.5772/55814

The majority of imprinted genes in mammals has a critical role in the development and function of the placenta [40] and brain [41], have been linked to cancer development and are associated with growth disorders, such as Beckwith-Wiedemann and Silver-Russel syndromes [42], and neurodevelopmental disorders, such as Angelman [43] and Prader-Willi syndromes [44].

3. Imprinting and cancer

Loss of imprinting (LOI), defined as the break the methylation patterns of DMRs associated with monoallelic parental-specific expression, is a common event in human cancer [45]. This term includes both the activation of the normally silenced allele and inactivation of the allele that is expressed upon normal imprinting conditions.

Abnormal imprinting of the *IGF2* and *H19* genes in tumors was first described in the Wilms' tumor [46,47]. This tumor is a common solid cancer in children, and loss of imprinting has been described as the most prevalent abnormality in the development of this tumor [48]. Thereafter, loss of imprinting of *IGF2* and *H19* genes has been correlated with several common adult human cancer (Table 1).

Despite these findings, the number of genes demonstrating LOI in human cancer is still limited due to the small number of known genes regulated by imprinting. However, the statistics may increase because of the growing interest in epigenetics and the large number of genes predicted to be regulated by imprinting.

Imprinted Gene	Oficial Name	Other Aliases	Chromosomal location	Cancer type	Reference
DIRAS3	DIRAS family, GTP-binding RAS-like 3	*ARHI, NOEY2*	1p31.1	Ovarian and breast	[49]
				Breast	[50]
				Myeloma	[51]
				Hepatocellular	[52,53]
				Thyroid	[54]
				Oligodendroglial	[55]
PLAGL1	pleiomorphic adenoma gene-like 1	*RP3-468K18.1, LOT1, ZAC, ZAC1*	6q24-q25	Breast and ovarian	[56]
				Gastric adenocarcinoma	[57]
				Cervical	[58]
PEG10	paternally expressed 10	*EDR, HB-1, MEF3L, Mar2, Mart2, RGAG3*	7q21	Hepatocellular	[59]
				B-cell chronic lymphocytic	[60]

Imprinted Gene	Oficial Name	Other Aliases	Chromosomal location	Cancer type	Reference
MEST	mesoderm specific transcript homolog (mouse)	*PEG1*	7q32	Osteossarcoma	[61]
				Lung	[62]
				Breast	[63]
				Uterine leiomyoma	[64]
				Wilms tumors	[65]
CDKN1C	cyclin-dependent kinase inhibitor 1C (p57, Kip2)	*BWCR, BWS, IMAGE, KIP2, WBS, p57*	11p15.5	Gastric	[66,67]
				Breast Lung	[68]
				Gastric Hepatocellular Pancreatic Acute myeloid leukemia	[69]
				Bladder	[70]
				Hepatocellular	[71]
				Rhabdoid	[72]
				Osteosarcoma	[61]
				Pancreatic ductal	[73]
				Esophageal	[74]
				Wilms	[75]
DLK1	delta-like 1 homolog (Drosophila)	*DLK, Delta1, FA1, PREF1, Pref-1, ZOG, pG2*	14q32.2	Hepatocellular	[76]
				Multiple myeloma	[77]
				Acute myeloid leukemia	[78]
PEG3	paternally expressed 3	*hCG_1685807, PW1, ZNF904, ZSCAN24*	19q13.4	Glioma	[79, 80]
				Ovarian	[81, 82]
NNAT	neuronatin	*Peg5*	20q11.2-q12	Pediatric acute leukemia	[83]
				Wilms	[65]
GNAS	GNAS complex locus	*RP4-543J19.4, AHO, C20orf45, GNAS1, GPSA, GSA, GSP, NESP, PHP1A, PHP1B, PHP1C, POH*	20q13.32	Pituitary	[84]
				Somatotroph adenomas	[85]
IGF2R	insulin-like growth factor 2 receptor	*CD222, CIMPR, M6P-R, MPR1, MPRI*	6q26	Wilms'tumor	[86]

Imprinted Gene	Oficial Name	Other Aliases	Chromosomal location	Cancer type	Reference
TFPI2	tissue factor pathway inhibitor 2	*PP5, REF1, TFPI-2*	7q22	Prostate	[87]
KCNQ1OT 1	KCNQ1 opposite strand/antisense transcript 1 (non-protein coding)	*KCNQ1-AS2, KCNQ10T1, KvDMR1, KvLQT1-AS, LIT1, NCRNA00012*	11p15	Colorectal	[88]
IGF2	insulin-like growth factor 2 (somatomedin A)	*PP1446, C11orf43, IGF-II, PP9974*	11p15.5	Gastric	[89]
				Hepatocellular	[90]
				Insulinomas	[91]
				Wilms' tumor	[92]
				Bladder	[93]
KCNQ1DN	KCNQ1 downstream neighbor (non-protein coding)	*BWRT; HSA404617*	11p15.5	Wilms' tumors	[94]
SLC22A18	solute carrier family 22, member 18	*BWR1A, BWSCR1A, HET, IMPT1, ITM, ORCTL2, SLC22A1L, TSSC5, p45-BWR1A*	11p15.5	Breast	[95]
WT1	Wilms tumor 1	*AWT1, EWS-WT1, GUD, NPHS4, WAGR, WIT-2, WT33*	11p13	Wilms' tumors	[96]
PEG3	paternally expressed 3	*hCG_1685807, PW1, ZNF904, ZSCAN24*	19q13.4	Glioma	[97, 98]
				Ovarian	[99]
H19	H19, imprinted maternally expressed transcript (non-protein coding)	*ASM, ASM1, BWS, D11S813E, LINC00008, NCRNA00008, PRO2605, WT2*	11p15.5	Colorectal	[100]
				Ovarian	[101]
				Hepatoblastoma	[102]
				Laryngeal squamous cell carcinoma	[103]
				Testicular seminomas	[104]
				Prostate	[105]
				Head and neck	[106]
				Ovarian	[101]
				Osteosarcoma	[107]
				Bladder	[108, 93]

Table 1. Imprinted genes and cancers with LOI and DNA-methylation changes.

4. Imprinting and bladder cancer

Bladder cancer is the second-most common genitourinary disorder and the sixth-most common disease in the world. Genetic and epigenetic alterations (Figure 1) are mostly likely involved in the malignant transformation and progression of this tumor type [109].

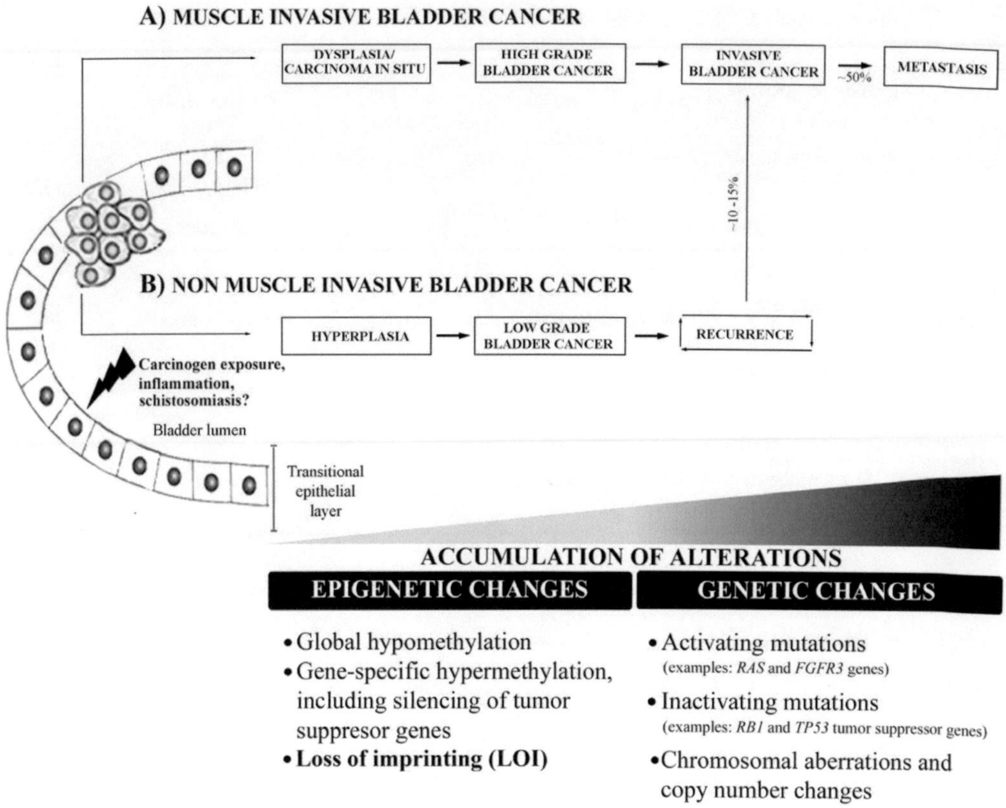

Figure 1. Urotherial carcinogenesis is a complex process resulting from the accumulation of genetic and epigenetic changes. Molecular and genetic analysis provide a framework for the characterization of molecular pathways (such as *RAS, FGFR3, RB1, TP53*-associated pathways) leading to tumor formation and clonal expansion. These pathways has been correlated with clinical and pathological parameters of both non-muscle and muscle invasive bladder cancer (A and B). Among other epigenetic changes, loss of imprinting (LOI) could lead to gene expression imbalances and contribute to the carcinogenesis process.

Currently, the diagnosis of bladder cancer is based on histological, pathological and morphological parameters and provides only a generalized outcome for patients [110]. In addition, the gold standard to detect and monitor bladder cancer is cystoscopy, which is an invasive and expensive method [111] even though this method shows poor performance in detecting low-grade tumors [112]. An understanding of cancer biomarkers will provide an opportunity to diagnose tumors earlier and with greater accuracy. Biomarkers can also help to identify those patients with a risk of disease recurrence, progression and metastasis as well as predict which tumors will respond to different therapeutic approaches [113].

Although there are numerous studies reporting aberrant DNA methylation of several tumor suppressor genes in bladder cancer, studies regarding LOI in this tumor type are sparse.

4.1. Catenin (cadherin-associated protein), alpha 3 gene — *CTNNA3*

The *CTNNA3* gene encodes a novel alpha-catenin, alphaT-catenin, that has related functions to alphaE-catenin, a well-known invasion suppressor gene necessary for the formation of cell-cell adhesion complexes. In support of the hypothesis that *CTNNA3* is a new imprinted gene, Oudejans *et al.* [114] demonstrated that the 10q21.3 region containing the *CTNNA3* gene shows parent-specific imprinting patterns and that the transcription of this gene is down-regulated in placental tissues of androgenetic origin. It was later demonstrated that the *CTNNA3* gene is subjected to imprinting in early placental tissues with preferential expression of the maternal allele in the first trimester placental tissues [115]. However, it was observed that *CTNNA3* imprinting depends on the trophoblast cell type because the expression in the extravillous trophoblast is biallelic, whereas the expression in villous cytotrophoblast is maternal and monoallelic. The expression of alphaT-catenin is also lost in villous syncytiotrophoblast as well as in extravillous trophoblast following epithelial-mesenchymal transition, similar to the imprinting pattern of the cyclin-dependent kinase inhibitor 1C (*CDKN1C*) gene, also known as p57KIP. Taken together, these findings suggest that both genes share a conserved regulatory mechanism that correlates with an early step in placental development.

To the best of our knowledge, there is only one report in the literature describing the frequency of monoallelic versus biallelic expression of *CTNNA3* in urothelial carcinomas of the bladder [116]. Approximately 35% of informative bladder cancers showed monoallelic expression, which was specifically associated with the tumor tissue. Furthermore, the *CTNNA3* transcript levels were significantly lower in tumor samples compared with the controls, all of which displayed biallelic expression. These data suggest that epigenetic alterations of *CTNNA3*, such as monoallelic expression, may disrupt key molecules involved in the protein interactions in adherens junctions, such as beta catenin and E-cadherin, making *CTNNA3* a candidate marker for disease progression.

4.2. Cyclin-dependent kinase inhibitor 1C gene — *CDKN1C*

In humans, the imprinted gene *CDKN1C* is located at 11p15.5. This gene is expressed from the maternally inherited allele and encodes the $p57^{KIP2}$ protein, an inhibitor of cyclin-dependent kinases. *CDKN1C* is considered a candidate tumor suppressor gene because of its location on a frequently deleted genomic region in human cancers, biochemical activities and imprinting regulation [117]. The imprinting of this locus is controlled by an ICR located ~ 700 kb from the *IGF2/H19* genes towards the centromere. The paternal allele of *CDKN1C* is silenced by the long non-coding *LIT1/KCNQ1OT1* RNA that originates from the differentially DNA-methylated KvDMR1 [11], where resides the promoter for this gene.

In bladder cancer, the down-regulation of *CDKN1C* can be explained by multiple mechanisms, including a switch of both alleles toward a paternal imprinting pattern as indicated by DMR hypomethylation and described by Hoffman *et al.* [70]. The other mechanisms proposed by the author include a loss of heterozygosity (loss of expression of the maternal allele) and the hypermethylation of the promoter region, although this mechanism cannot be the only one responsible for the down-regulation of *CDKN1C*. Other studies have indicated that *CDKN1C* is a putative tumor suppressor gene in bladder cancer due to the reduced mRNA and protein levels compared with normal tissue. By immunohistochemical analysis, it was observed that the presence of the $p57^{KIP2}$ protein was detected in only 25.8% of the samples but in 100% of normal urinary bladder mucosa [118] suggesting that a decrease in $p57^{KIP2}$ expression may be a biomarker for bladder cancer. Furthermore, the decreased expression of *CDKN1C* mRNA was frequently observed in a study using samples of urothelial carcinoma tissues and cell lines. Interestingly, loss of *CDKN1C* transcripts was correlated with the loss of *H19* mRNA expression [119].

4.3. *H19*-imprinted maternally expressed transcript (non-protein coding) / insulin-like growth factor gene (*IFG2*)

The *IGF2* and *H19* genes are located in the human chromosome at 11p15.5. The imprinted cluster in this region has been implicated in a variety of cancers. Initially, the *H19* gene was thought to be involved in human cancer because of its potential tumor suppressor activity. When tumor cell lines were transformed with an expression vector containing this gene, there were morphological changes and a delay of growth [120]. However, later studies suggested that the *H19* gene has oncofetal characteristics due to abundant expression in some human fetal tissues and tumors arising from these tissues [121].

Although the mechanism of *H19* activity is controversial, it has been shown that the expression patterns of several genes are altered in the presence of *H19* RNA expression. These genes have been linked to potentially malignant cellular processes such as invasion, migration and angiogenesis. Additionally, the expression of some genes with functions in cell adhesion was inversely correlated with *H19* expression, which may lead to the development of more invasive tumors [122].

The *H19* gene produces a 2.3-kb non-coding RNA transcript that is capped, spliced and polyadenylated. No protein product has been identified. Recently, Cai and Cullen [123] showed that the *H19* transcript can function as a primary miRNA in humans and mice. These authors suggested that although this miR-675 is a derivative of the *H19* gene, it does not have a defined role, although it is possible that it functions as a regulator of mRNAs.

The *IGF2* gene encodes the insulin-like growth factor II protein, which is structurally homologous to insulin, and promotes growth and plays a role in metabolic processes in various cell types [45]. *IGF2* is regulated in a precise manner to maintain the monoallelic expression, which highlights the importance of gene dosage. The LOI of *IGF2* was first observed in the Wilms' tumor [46, 47], and subsequent studies have found that aberrant imprinting or LOI of *IGF2* is linked to many types of tumors.

Investigation into the role of the *H19* in bladder cancer began in 1995. Ariel *et al.* [121] suggested that the *H19* gene was a potential cancer marker because it was prominently expressed in more malignant and invasive transitional cell carcinomas as well as in *in situ* carcinomas, demonstrating unpredictable behavior with high rates of recurrence, progression and metastasis. These data were later confirmed, demonstrating that *H19* expression was specifically associated with tumors, with no detection of expression in normal urinary bladder mucosa, suggesting that *H19* may have oncogenic properties in the bladder urothelium [124].

Disrupted *H19* imprinting was first demonstrated in bladder cancer in a small number of samples. Among the four informative samples (heterozygotes for a neutral genetic polymorphism), two tumors showed biallelic expression of the *H19* gene. The same study showed LOI of the *IGF2* gene in three cases [93]. LOI of *IGF2* and *H19* at low frequencies was also described by another study in which only 12.5% and 22.2% of informative samples for the *H19* and *IGF2* genes, respectively, demonstrated this alteration. A DNA methylation analysis of the DMR showed a consistent decrease in the percentage of methylation from normal to tumoral tissue in the methylated allele. In both the methylated and unmethylated alleles of the *IGF2* DMR, the average amount of methylation decreased from normal to tumoral bladder tissue, showing a relationship between the altered methylation in the DMR and a loss of imprinting pattern in bladder cancer [125].

Most tumors in the urinary bladder are superficial, with a low risk of metastasis. In less than one third of the cases, the tumor is invasive and compromises the muscle layer. Despite this low risk of metastasis, bladder cancer has a high risk of recurrence [126]. The *IGF2* gene was shown to have a role in invasion and metastasis in several types of cancer (reviewed in [127]. In bladder cancer, a recent study showed a connection between the increased levels of *IGF2* and cytoplasmic immunolocalization of E-cadherin in nonmuscle invasive tumors with 57% of analyzed tumors demonstrating LOI and cytoplasmic expression of E-cadherin. The study also demonstrated that E-cadherin may indicate tumor recurrence independently of tumor grade or stage [128]. The *CDH1* gene encodes a critical protein involved in epithelial adhesion. The process of epithelial-mesenchymal transition (EMT) has been identified as an important prognostic biomarker in bladder cancer [129] and plays a central role in the process of carcinoma cell dispersion [130]. Morali *et al.* [131] demonstrated that the IGF2 protein induced the spread and loss of cell-cell contacts in rat bladder carcinomas derived from NBT-II cells and decreased the mean tumor height from 6.8 μm to 4 μm after 3 hours of treatment with IGF2.

The ICR located upstream of the *H19* gene and its DMR contains seven CTCF binding sites. Takai *et al.* [108] analyzed these sites in normal human embryonic ureteral tissue and found that only the sixth site demonstrated allele-specific methylation, whereas the others sites were methylated. In the analysis of the sixth site in six samples of human bladder cancer, two cases showed hypomethylation of the paternal allele, and the CpG islands in the maternal alleles of the remaining cases were sporadically methylated. The methylation status of the sixth CTCF-binding site was also investigated in human bladder cancer and normal bladder tissues. The authors suggested that the hypomethylation of the paternal allele observed in bladder cancer was nearly absent in normal bladder tissue. This hypomethylation could be more prevalent than methylation in the maternal allele at this locus and might play a role in the overexpression of *H19* in advanced-stage bladder cancer, as reported by Cooper *et al.* [124].

Carcinogen exposure is one of the mechanisms implicated in the development of human bladder carcinomas. In a mouse study that induced bladder cancer by N-butyl-N-(4-hydro-butyl) nitrosamine exposure, the expression of *H19* was first noted in the lamina propria (the drug was administered for 5 weeks) and posteriorly in epithelial cells (the drug was administered for 20-28 weeks). The alterations in *H19* expression levels were consistent with preneoplastic changes in the transitional epithelium of the bladder [132].

Because the *H19* gene is not expressed (or is expressed at low levels) in normal adult tissues but is expressed in tumors derived from tissues previously expressing it during the embryogenic period, *H19* could be exploited for alternative therapeutic approaches. In fact, regulatory sequences of *H19* were used in a vector that expressed diphtheria toxin (DT-A) or herpes simplex virus thymidine kinase (HSV-tk) that were then transfected into tumoral cell lines, including a cell line derived from bladder cancer, and injected in an animal model of bladder cancer. It was found that the expression of DT-A was specific to T24P bladder cancer cells compared with human fibroblast IMR-90 cells. The in vivo experiment showed that the weights of the tumors from DTA-PBH19-treated animals (with 3 doses) were significantly less than the tumors from the control animals. Similar results were observed in animals treated with the *TK-H19* construct and ganciclovir (GCV) in a single dose, although the tumors started to resist the growth-inhibitory effects of the *TK-PBH19* and GCV treatment after the eighth day of treatment. These initial findings demonstrated that the *H19* regulatory sequence was capable of driving expression of therapeutic genes [133].

Recently, a double promoter expressing DT-A was constructed with two regulatory sequences (*H19* and *IGF2*-P4) and tested in bladder cancer cell lines and animal models. The inclusion of two promoters was more efficient at lysing the cancer cell lines when compared to the single-promoter constructs, *H19*-DTA or *IGF2*-DTA. This increased efficacy was also observed in the growth inhibition of heterotopic bladder tumors, with a 70% reduction in tumor development compared to controls after three injections. The treatment of orthotopic tumors inhibited tumor growth, reducing the size of treated tumors to 86% of the size of tumors found in the control animals [134]. These findings suggest that this approach could be applied in cancer therapy.

4.4. Predict imprinted genes and bladder cancer

Although few studies have reported LOI in well characterized imprinted genes (such as *IGF2* and *H19*) in bladder cancer, there is a list of newly predicted imprinted genes already implicated in this type of tumor, some of them are candidates to diagnostic and/or prognosis markers.

A newly identified gene, *BLCAP* (bladder cancer associated protein), is a novel tumor suppressor gene candidate in human bladder cancer. This gene, also known as BC10 protein (bladder cancer-10 kDa protein), is located at 20q11.23 and encodes a small protein with unknown cellular functions. Although it has no homology to any known protein [135], it includes putative cytoplasmic domains at the N- and C-terminal ends, a SPXX motif and a

http://dx.doi.org/10.5772/55814

proline-rich area resembling the PXXP domain, which suggests that it may play a role in cell signaling [136]. Transcriptional down-regulation of this gene has been observed in different tumor types [137-138-139] including invasive bladder cancer [136]. In support of its role as a tumor suppressor, Fan *et al.* [140] showed that overexpression of *BLCAP* resulted in growth inhibition and induced apoptosis of human Ewing's sarcoma cells *in vitro*. In a recent study of 120 patients and validated with 2,108 samples, the authors confirmed that the loss of *BLCAP* expression is associated with tumor progression, high levels of nuclear protein expression and a poor prognosis, suggesting that *BLCAP* expression may be a prognostic biomarker[135].

BLCAP was initially considered a non-imprinted gene in human fetal tissues, with biallelic expression in the fetal brain, adrenal gland, heart, kidney, liver, lung and placental tissues, and showed an unmethylated promoter-associated CpG island in all tissues evaluated [141]. Recently, it was demonstrated that the *BLCAP* gene is imprinted in the human and mouse brains and this tissue-specific pattern may be regulated by the high levels of *NNAT* transcription in the brain [142]. The *NNAT* gene lies within the intron of the *BLCAP* gene [142] and is specifically expressed from the paternal allele in the central nervous system from mid-gestation through early postnatal development [141]. Since that *NNAT* gene may influences the imprinting of the *BLCAP* gene, it may be interesting to study the loss of imprinting of both genes in bladder cancer.

Another gene that may be regulated by genomic imprinting is the retinoblastoma tumor susceptibility gene (*RB1*). This important discovery was made in a genome-wide analysis of CpG methylation from the blood sample of a child with multiple imprinting defects. This study revealed a differential methylation pattern of a specific CpG island located within the intron 2 of the *RB1* gene. It was suggested that the presence of the CpG island resulted from a retrotransposition event in the KIAA0649 gene between exon 4 and an 18 bp segment of the 3′end of exon 3. The authors also showed that the CpG island 85 is unmethylated on the paternal chromosome and that this CpG island on the maternal chromosome is methylated, with a difference in gene expression favoring the maternal allele [143]. This finding was unexpected because the paternal transcripts were predicted to be more highly expressed than the maternal transcripts. According to the authors, this finding could be a result of transcriptional interference in which the lack of methylation of CpG number 85 and the expression of a transcript (2B-transcript) could interfere with the expression of the paternal allele. To explain this finding, Buiting *et al.* [144] proposed a model in which the binding of a transcriptional complex in the unmethylated 2B-promoter region (paternal) blocks the transcriptional complex that regulates the expression of an alternate transcript from the promoter located upstream to exon 1, resulting in a low abundance of the paternal allele. Recently, Nakabayashi *et al.* [145] confirmed the maternal methylation of the RB1 DMR in a study of rare reciprocal genome-wide uniparental disomy samples in patients with Beckwith–Wiedemann and Silver–Russell syndrome-like phenotypes.

The *RB1* gene was one of the first tumor suppressor genes discovered, and its loss of function has been reported in various tumor types. Rb1 protein interacts with a large and steadily growing list of cellular proteins and an even greater number of genes [146], reinforcing its central role in carcinogenesis. In bladder cancer, there are a large number of studies implicating the *RB1* gene in tumoral development and progression. Aggressive tumoral behavior, such as in invasive high-stage muscle tumors, was associated with the down-regulation of *RB1* mRNA and protein in addition to altered mRNA expression of *TP16* and *CDK4* [147].

In some regions in the world, bladder cancer is associated with the urinary form of schistosomiasis. Abdulamir *et al.* [148] profiled the molecular markers in schistosomal and non-schistosomal bladder tumors and found lower expression levels of Rb protein in patient tumors not caused by parasitic infection and an association between down-regulation of the protein and late stages of the disease (III and IV) in the schistosomal and invasive non-schistosomal bladder tumors. These findings support the hypothesis that the Rb protein can be used as a prognostic marker and distinguish a tumor caused by infection from a tumor not caused by infection.

According to the model proposed by Buiting *et al.* [144], the loss of imprinting (demethylation of the maternal allele) could explain the lack/decrease in *RB1* gene transcripts mentioned above, highlighting the need to understand the mechanisms behind the down-regulation of the *RB1* gene. Furthermore, methylation of the RB1 gene promoter was evaluated in 45 patients with bladder cancer and in bladder cancer cell lines. However, the authors found unmethylated promoter-associated CpG island in all bladder cancer cell lines and primary tumors examined [149]. More recently, a study involving a large number of genes investigated the methylation status of 25 proven or suspected tumor suppressor genes in pT1G3 transitional cell carcinomas. The authors found that tumors displaying unmethylated *RB1* and *TP73*, among others genes, had higher progression rates in patients treated with non-maintenance bacillus Calmette-Guérion (BCG) [150].

These studies found an unexpected result compared with the studies of *RB1* gene expression, as the decreased expression of this gene could be linked to hypermethylation of the promoter. However, these studies did not examine the expression of the *RB1* gene; therefore, the association between the unmethylated promoter and cancer progression found in the study by Agundez *et al.* [150] could be due to the decreased expression of the gene associated with a loss of imprinting (demethylated maternal allele) at intronic CpG island 85.

TP73 is a *TP53*-related gene that encodes a p73 protein that shares considerable homology with the tumor suppressor gene *TP53*, which was previously associated with the development of neuroblastoma and other tumors [151]. This gene is located at 1p36.3 and was shown to be a monoallelically expressed gene (reviewed in [152]) with maternal expression. Information about the imprinting of *TP73* gene in cancers is still limited and contradictory [153]. Kaghad *et al.* [151] demonstrated that p73 is a candidate for the putative, imprinted neuroblastoma suppressor gene; however, studies have shown a relationship between the loss of imprinting (biallelic expression and switching alleles) and some types of cancer, such as ovarian cancer [154], breast cancer [155] and gastric adenocarcinoma [156].

In bladder cancer, the loss of imprinting and an elevated expression of the *TP73* gene was suggested at first by Chi *et al.* [157], who found *TP73* biallelic expression in 52.2% of tumor samples analyzed but not in the normal tissue samples, with higher expression of the transcript in biallelic expressers (66.7%), whereas only 2 (18.2%) of 11 monoallelic expressers showed

http://dx.doi.org/10.5772/55814

high expression levels of this transcript. The authors also demonstrated that there is a positive correlation between high expression of *TP73* and tumor stage or grade. Based on these findings, it was suggested that the *TP73* gene is not a tumor suppressor in bladder carcinogenesis and that the loss of imprinting (activation of a silent allele) could contribute to the progression of bladder tumors. The overexpression of the *TP73* was also observed in 22 of 23 bladder cancer samples in a second study. However, when the allele-specific expression was evaluated, the biallelic expression of the gene was observed in all cancers and matched normal tissues [158].

5. Perspectives

It is well known that disruption of epigenetic processes can lead to altered gene expression associated with malignant cellular transformation. Still, it has been demonstrated that LOI occurs in a large variety of human cancers, however it remains to be determined if there is a commonality to the cell type which initially undergoes this alteration [159]. Moreover there is a need for greater knowledge of imprinted genes, since disrupted expression of them has been shown to have either oncogenic or tumour suppressing activity [11]. Future studies will provide new insights, particularly into interactions between products of imprinted genes in physiological pathways [9]. Among other epigenetic changes, the loss of imprinting in cancer may prove useful for advancing our knowledge and for development of new prognostic and therapeutic biomarkers.

Author details

Mariana Bisarro dos Reis and Cláudia Aparecida Rainho

Department of Genetics, Institute of Biosciences, Sao Paulo State University – UNESP, Botucatu – Sao Paulo, Brazil

References

[1] Lim DH, Maher ER. Genomic imprinting syndromes and cancer. Advances in Genetics 2010; 70:145-75.

[2] Barlow DP. Genomic imprinting: a mammalian epigenetic discovery model. Annual Review of Genetics 2011; 45: 379-403.

[3] Hayward BE, Moran V, Strain L, Bonthron DT. Bidirectional imprinting of a single gene: *GNAS1* encodes maternally, paternally, and biallelically derived proteins. Proceedings of the National Academy of Sciences 1998; 95: 15475–15480.

[4] www.geneimprint.com/site/genes-by-species. Access in 06/08/12.

[5] Ferguson-Smith AC. Genomic imprinting: the emergence of an epigenetic paradigm. Nature Review Genetics 2011; 12(8): 565-575.

[6] Ioshikhes IP, Zhang MQ. Large-scale human promoter mapping using CpG islands. Nature Genetics 2000; 26: 61–63.

[7] Kaneda M, Okano M, Hata K, Sado T, Tsujimoto N, Li E, Sasaki H. Essential role for de novo DNA methyltransferase Dnmt3a in paternal and maternal imprinting. Nature 2004, 429: 900-903.

[8] Morgan HD, Santos F, Green K, Dean W, Reik W. Epigenetic reprogramming in mammals. Human Molecular Genetics 2005; 14(1): R47-R58.

[9] Reik W, Walter J. Genomic imprinting: parental influence on the genome. Nature Review Genetics 2001; 2(1): 21-32.

[10] Bartolomei MS. Genomic imprinting: employing and avoiding epigenetic processes. Genes & Development 2009; 23(18): 2124-2133.

[11] Monk D. Deciphering the cancer imprintome. Briefings in Functional Genomics 2010; 9(4): 329-339.

[12] Verona RI, Mann MR and Bartolomei MS. Genomic imprinting: Intricacies of epigenetic regulation in clusters. Annual Review of Cell and Developmental Biology 2003; 19: 237–259.

[13] Wan LB, Bartolomei MS. Regulation of imprinting in clusters: noncoding RNAs versus insulators. Advances in Genetics 2008; 61: 207-223.

[14] Ideraabdullah FY, Vigneau S, Bartolomei MS. Genomic imprinting mechanisms in mammals. Mutation Research 2008; 647(1-2): 77-85.

[15] Bhaumik SR, Smith E, Shilatifard A. Covalent modifications of histones during development and disease pathogenesis. Nature Structural & Molecular Biology. 2007; 14: 1008–1016.

[16] Kouzarides T. Chromatin modifications and their function. Cell 2007; 128: 693–705.

[17] Arnaud P. Genomic imprinting in germ cells: imprints are under control. Reproduction 2010; 140(3): 411-423.

[18] Delaval K, Govin J, Cerqueira F, Rousseaux S, Khochbin S, Feil R. Differential histone modifications mark mouse imprinting control regions during spermatogenesis. The EMBO Journal 2007; 26(3): 720-729.

[19] Black JC, Whetstine JR. Chromatin landscape: methylation beyond transcription. Epigenetics 2011; 6(1): 9-15.

[20] Henckel A, Nakabayashi K, Sanz LA, Feil R, Hata K, Arnaud P. Histone methylation is mechanistically linked to DNA methylation at imprinting control regions in mammals. Human Molecular Genetics 2009; 18(18): 3375-3383.

[21] Zhang Y, Tycko, B. Monoallelic expression of the human *H19* gene. Nature Genetics 1992; 1: 40-44.

[22] Lewis A, Murrell, A. Genomic imprinting: CTCF protects the boundaries. Current Biology 2004; 14(7): 284-286.

[23] Leighton PA, Saam JR, Ingram RS, Stewart CL, Tilghman SM. An enhancer deletion affects both *H19* and *IFG2* expression. Genes & Development 1995; 9(17): 2079-2089.

[24] Kaffer CR, Srivastava M, Park KY, Ives E, Hsieh S, Batlle J, Grinberg A, Huang SP, Pfeifer K. A transcriptional insulator at the imprinted *H19* /*IFG2* locus. Genes & Development 2000; 14(15): 1908-1919.

[25] Tremblay KD, Duran KL, Bartolomei MS A 5' 2-kilobase-pair region of the imprinted mouse *H19* gene exhibits exclusive paternal methylation throughout development. Molecular Cell Biology 1997; 17(8): 4322-4329.

[26] Bell AC, Felsenfeld G. Methylation of a CTCF-dependent boundary controls imprinted expression of the *IFG2* gene. Nature 2000; 405(6785): 482-485.

[27] Pan Y, He B, Li T, Zhu C, Zhang L, Wang B, Xu Y, Qu L, Hoffman AR, Wang S, Hu J. Targeted tumor gene therapy based on loss of *IGF2* imprinting. Cancer Biology and Therapy 2010; 10(3): 290-298.

[28] Bartolomei MS, Ferguson-Smith AC. Mammalian genomic imprinting. Cold Spring Harbor Perspectives in Biology 2011; 3(7) pii: a002592.

[29] Yang J, Corces VG. Chromatin insulators: a role in nuclear organization and gene expression. Advances in Cancer Research 2011; 110: 43-76.

[30] Murrell A, Heeson S, Reik W. Interaction between differentially methylated regions partitions the imprinted genes *IFG2* and *H19* into parent-specific chromatin loops. Nature Genetics 2004; 36(8): 889-893.

[31] Kurukuti S, Tiwari VK, Tavoosidana G, Pugacheva E, Murrell A, Zhao Z, Lobanenkov V, Reik W, Ohlsson R. CTCF binding at the *H19* imprinting control region mediates maternally inherited higher-order chromatin conformation to restrict enhancer access to *IFG2*. Proceedings of the National Academy of Sciences of the United States of America 2006; 103(28): 10684-10689.

[32] Engel N, Raval AK, Thorvaldsen JL, Bartolomei SM. Three-dimensional conformation at the *H19*/*IFG2* locus supports a model of enhancer tracking. Human Molecular Genetics 2008; 17(19): 3021-3029.

[33] Malecová B, Morris KV. Transcriptional gene silencing through epigenetic changes mediated by non-coding RNAs. Current Opinion in Molecular Therapeutics 2010; 12(2): 214-222.

[34] Royo H, Cavaillé J. Non-coding RNAs in imprinted gene clusters. Biology of the Cell 2008; 100(3): 149-166.

[35] Zhou H, Hu H, Lai M. Non-coding RNAs and their epigenetic regulatory mechanisms. Biology of the Cell 2010; 102(12): 645-655.

[36] Braidotti G, Baubec T, Pauler F, Seidl C, Smrzka O, Stricker S, Yotova I, Barlow DP. The Air noncoding RNA: an imprinted cis-silencing transcript. Cold Spring Harbor Symposia on Quantitative Biology 2004; 69: 55–66.

[37] Seidl CI, Stricker SH, Barlow DP. The imprinted Air ncRNA is an atypical RNAPII transcript that evades splicing and escapes nuclear export. The EMBO Journal 2006; 25(15): 3565–3575.

[38] Shin JY, Fitzpatrick GV, Higgins MJ. Two distinct mechanisms of silencing by the KvDMR1 imprinting control region. The EMBO Journal 2008; 27(1): 168-178.

[39] Hore TA, Rapkins RW, Graves JA. Construction and evolution of imprinted loci in mammals. Trends in Genetics 2007; 23(9): 440-448.

[40] Piedrahita JA. The role of imprinted genes in fetal growth abnormalities. Birth Defects Research. Part A, Clinical and Molecular Teratology 2011; 91(8): 682-692.

[41] Davies W, Isles AR, Humby T, Wilkinson LS. What are imprinted genes doing in the brain? Epigenetics 2007; 2(4): 201-206.

[42] Nativio R, Sparago A, Ito Y, Weksberg R, Riccio A, Murrell A. Disruption of genomic neighbourhood at the imprinted *IFG2 -H19* locus in Beckwith-Wiedemann syndrome and Silver-Russell syndrome. Human Molecular Genetics 2011; 20(7): 1363-1374.

[43] Mabb AM, Judson MC, Zylka MJ, Philpot BD. Angelman syndrome: insights into genomic imprinting and neurodevelopmental phenotypes. Trends in Neurosciences 2011; 34(6): 293-303.

[44] Hirasawa R, Feil R. Genomic imprinting and human disease. Essays in Biochemistry 2010; 48(1): 187-200.

[45] Cui H. Loss of imprinting of *IGF2* as an epigenetic marker for the risk of human cancer. Disease Markers 2007; 23(1-2): 105-112.

[46] Ogawa O, Eccles MR, Szeto J, McNoe LA, Yun K, Maw MA, Smith PJ, Reeve AE. Relaxation of insulin-like growth factor II gene imprinting implicated in Wilms' tumour Nature 1993; 362(6422): 749-751.

[47] Rainier S, Johnson LA, Dobry CJ, Ping AJ, Grundy PE, Feinberg AP. Relaxation of imprinted genes in human cancer Nature 1993; 362(6422): 747-749.

[48] Feinberg AP, Cui H, Ohlsson R.DNA methylation and genomic imprinting: insights from cancer into epigenetic mechanisms. Seminars in Cancer Biology 2002; 12(5): 389-398.

[49] Yu Y, Luo R, Lu Z, Wei Feng W, Badgwell D, Issa JP, Rosen DG, Liu J, Bast RC Jr. Biochemistry and biology of ARHI (D53]IRAS3), an imprinted tumor suppressor gene whose expression is lost in ovarian and breast cancers. Methods in Enzymology 2006; 407: 455-468.

[50] Yuan J, Luo RZ, Fujii S, Wang L, Hu W, Andreeff M, Pan Y, Kadota M, Oshimura M, Sahin AA, Issa JP, Bast RC Jr, Yu Y. Aberrant methylation and silencing of ARHI, an imprinted tumor suppressor gene in which the function is lost in breast cancers. Cancer Research 2003; 63(14): 4174-4180.

[51] Ria R, Todoerti K, Berardi S, Coluccia AM, De Luisi A, Mattioli M, Ronchetti D, Morabito F, Guarini A, Petrucci MT, Dammacco F, Ribatti D, Neri A, Vacca A. Gene expression profiling of bone marrow endothelial cells in patients with multiple myeloma. Clinical Cancer Research 2009; 15(17): 5369-5378.

[52] Huang J, Lin Y, Li L, Qing D, Teng XM, Zhang YL, Hu X, Hu Y, Yang P, Han ZG. ARHI, as a novel suppressor of cell growth and downregulated in human hepatocellular carcinoma, could contribute to hepatocarcinogenesis. Molecular Carcinogenesis 2009; 48(2): 130-140.

[53] Zhao X, Li J, Zhuo J, Cai L.Reexpression of ARHI inhibits tumor growth and angiogenesis and impairs the mTOR/VEGF pathway in hepatocellular carcinoma. Biochemical and Biophysical Research Communications 2010; 403(3-4): 417-421.

[54] Weber F, Aldred MA, Morrison CD, Plass C, Frilling A, Broelsch CE, Waite KA, Eng C Silencing of the maternally imprinted tumor suppressor ARHI contributes to follicular thyroid carcinogenesis The Journal of Clinical Endocrinology & Metabolism 2005; 90(2): 1149-1155.

[55] Riemenschneider MJ, Reifenberger J, Reifenberger G. Frequent biallelic inactivation and transcriptional silencing of the DIRAS3 gene at 1p31 in oligodendroglial tumors with 1p loss. International Journal of Cancer 2008; 122(11): 2503-2510.

[56] Abdollahi A, Pisarcik D, Roberts D, Weinstein J, Cairns P, Hamilton TC. LOT1 (PLAGL1/ZAC1), the candidate tumor suppressor gene at chromosome 6q24-25, is epigenetically regulated in cancer. The Journal of Biological Chemistry 2003; 278(8): 6041-6049.

[57] Leal MF, Lima EM, Silva PN, Assumpção PP, Calcagno DQ, Payão SL, Burbano RR, Smith MA. Promoter hypermethylation of CDH1, FHIT, MTAP and PLAGL1 in gastric adenocarcinoma in individuals from Northern Brazil. World Journal of Gastroenterology 2007; 13(18): 2568-2574.

[58] Song JY, Lee JK, Lee NW, Jung HH, Kim SH, Lee KW. Microarray analysis of normal cervix, carcinoma in situ, and invasive cervical cancer: identification of candidate

genes in pathogenesis of invasion in cervical cancer. International Journal of Gynecological Cancer 2008; 18(5): 1051-1059.

[59] Wang C, Xiao Y, Hu Z, Chen Y, Liu N, Hu G *PEG10* directly regulated by E2Fs might have a role in the development of hepatocellular carcinoma. FEBS Letters 2008; 582(18): 2793-2798.

[60] Kainz B, Shehata M, Bilban M, Kienle D, Heintel D, Krömer-Holzinger E, Le T, Kröber A, Heller G, Schwarzinger I, Demirtas D, Chott A, Döhner H, Zöchbauer-Müller S, Fonatsch C, Zielinski C, Stilgenbauer S, Gaiger A, Wagner O, Jäger U.Overexpression of the paternally expressed gene 10 (PEG10) from the imprinted locus on chromosome 7q21 in high-risk B-cell chronic lymphocytic leukemia. International Journal of Cancer 2007; 121(9): 1984-1993.

[61] Li Y, Meng G, Guo QN.Changes in genomic imprinting and gene expression associated with transformation in a model of human osteosarcoma. Experimental and Molecular Pathology 2008; 84(3): 234-239.

[62] Nakanishi H, Suda T, Katoh M, Watanabe A, Igishi T, Kodani M, Matsumoto S, Nakamoto M, Shigeoka Y, Okabe T, Oshimura M, Shimizu E. Loss of imprinting of PEG1/MEST in lung cancer cell lines. Oncology Reports 2004; 12(6): 1273-1278.

[63] Pedersen IS, Dervan PA, Broderick D, Harrison M, Miller N, Delany E, O'Shea D, Costello P, McGoldrick A, Keating G, Tobin B, Gorey T, McCann A.Frequent loss of imprinting of PEG1/MEST in invasive breast cancer. Cancer Research 1999; 59(21): 5449-5451.

[64] Moon YS, Park SK, Kim HT, Lee TS, Kim JH, Choi YS.Imprinting and expression status of isoforms 1 and 2 of PEG1/MEST gene in uterine leiomyoma. Gynecologic and Obstetric Investigation 2010; 70(2): 120-125.

[65] Hubertus J, Lacher M, Rottenkolber M, Müller-Höcker J, Berger M, Stehr M, von Schweinitz D, Kappler R. Altered expression of imprinted genes in Wilms tumors. Oncology Reports 2011; 25(3): 817-823.

[66] Shin JY, Kim HS, Lee KS, Kim J, Park JB, Won MH, Chae SW, Choi YH, Choi KC, Park YE, Lee JY Mutation and expression of the p27KIP1 and p57KIP2 genes in human gastric cancer. Experimental and Molecular Medicine 2000; 32(2): 79-83.

[67] Liang B, Wang S, Yang X, Ye Y, Yu Y, Cui Z.Expressions of cyclin E, cyclin dependent kinase 2 and p57(KIP2) in human gastric cancer. Chinese Medical Journal (English Edition) 2003; 116(1): 20-23.

[68] Kobatake T, Yano M, Toyooka S, Tsukuda K, Dote H, Kikuchi T, Toyota M, Ouchida M, Aoe M, Date H, Pass HI, Doihara H, Shimizu N.Aberrant methylation of p57KIP2 gene in lung and breast cancers and malignant mesotheliomas. Oncology Reports 2004; 12(5): 1087-1092.

[69] Kikuchi T, Toyota M, Itoh F, Suzuki H, Obata T, Yamamoto H, Kakiuchi H, Kusano M, Issa JP, Tokino T, Imai K. Inactivation of p57KIP2 by regional promoter hyperme-

thylation and histone deacetylation in human tumors. Oncogene 2002; 21(17): 2741-2749.

[70] Hoffmann MJ, Florl AR, Seifert HH, Schulz WA Multiple mechanisms downregulate CDKN1C in human bladder cancer. International Journal of Cancer 2005; 114(3): 406-413.

[71] Schwienbacher C, Gramantieri L, Scelfo R, Veronese A, Calin GA, Bolondi L, Croce CM, Barbanti-Brodano G, Negrini M.Gain of imprinting at chromosome 11p15: A pathogenetic mechanism identified in human hepatocarcinomas. Proceedings of the National Academy of Sciences 2000; 97(10): 5445-5449.

[72] Algar EM, Muscat A, Dagar V, Rickert C, Chow CW, Biegel JA, Ekert PG, Saffery R, Craig J, Johnstone RW, Ashley DM. Imprinted CDKN1C is a tumor suppressor in rhabdoid tumor and activated by restoration of SMARCB1 and histone deacetylase inhibitors. PLoS One 2009; 4(2): e4482.

[73] Sato N, Matsubayashi H, Abe T, Fukushima N, Goggins M. Epigenetic down-regulation of CDKN1C/p57KIP2 in pancreatic ductal neoplasms identified by gene expression profiling. Clinical Cancer Research 2005; 11(13): 4681-4688.

[74] Soejima H, Nakagawachi T, Zhao W, Higashimoto K, Urano T, Matsukura S, Kitajima Y, Takeuchi M, Nakayama M, Oshimura M, Miyazaki K, Joh K, Mukai T. Silencing of imprinted CDKN1C gene expression is associated with loss of CpG and histone H3 lysine 9 methylation at DMR-LIT1 in esophageal cancer. Oncogene 2004; 23(25): 4380-4388.

[75] Schwienbacher C, Angioni A, Scelfo R, Veronese A, Calin GA, Massazza G, Hatada I, Barbanti-Brodano G, Negrini M.Abnormal RNA expression of 11p15 imprinted genes and kidney developmental genes in Wilms' tumor. Cancer Research 2000; 60(6): 1521-1525.

[76] Huang J, Zhang X, Zhang M, Zhu JD, Zhang YL, Lin Y, Wang KS, Qi XF, Zhang Q, Liu GZ, Yu J, Cui Y, Yang PY, Wang ZQ, Han ZG. Up-regulation of DLK1 as an imprinted gene could contribute to human hepatocellular carcinoma. Carcinogenesis 2007; 28(5): 1094-1103.

[77] Benetatos L, Dasoula A, Hatzimichael E, Georgiou I, Syrrou M, Bourantas KL. Promoter hypermethylation of the MEG3 (DLK1/MEG3) imprinted gene in multiple myeloma. Clinical Lymphoma Myeloma and Leukemia 2008; 8(3): 171-175.

[78] Khoury H, Suarez-Saiz F, Wu S, Minden MD. An upstream insulator regulates DLK1 imprinting in AML. Blood 2010; 115(11): 2260-2263.

[79] Jiang X, Yu Y, Yang HW, Agar NY, Frado L, Johnson MD. The imprinted gene PEG3 inhibits Wnt signaling and regulates glioma growth. The Journal of Biological Chemistry 2010; 285(11): 8472-8480.

[80] Otsuka S, Maegawa S, Takamura A, Kamitani H, Watanabe T, Oshimura M, Nanba E. Aberrant promoter methylation and expression of the imprinted PEG3 gene in

glioma. Proceedings of the Japan Academy - Series B: Physical & Biological Sciences 2009; 85(4): 157-165.

[81] Feng W, Marquez RT, Lu Z, Liu J, Lu KH, Issa JP, Fishman DM, Yu Y, Bast RC Jr. Imprinted tumor suppressor genes ARHI and PEG3 are the most frequently down-regulated in human ovarian cancers by loss of heterozygosity and promoter methylation. Cancer 2008; 112(7): 1489-1502.

[82] Dowdy SC, Gostout BS, Shridhar V, Wu X, Smith DI, Podratz KC, Jiang SW. Biallelic methylation and silencing of paternally expressed gene 3 (PEG3) in gynecologic cancer cell lines. Gynecologic Oncology 2005; 99(1): 126-134.

[83] Kuerbitz SJ, Pahys J, Wilson A, Compitello N, Gray TA. Hypermethylation of the imprinted NNAT locus occurs frequently in pediatric acute leukemia. Carcinogenesis 2002; 23(4): 559-564.

[84] Mantovani G, Lania AG, Spada A. GNAS imprinting and pituitary tumors. Molecular and Cellular Endocrinology 2010; 326(1-2): 15-18.

[85] Picard C, Silvy M, Gerard C, Buffat C, Lavaque E, Figarella-Branger D, Dufour H, Gabert J, Beckers A, Brue T, Enjalbert A, Barlier A. Gs alpha overexpression and loss of Gs alpha imprinting in human somatotroph adenomas: association with tumor size and response to pharmacologic treatment. International Journal of Cancer 2007; 121(6): 1245-1252.

[86] Xu YQ, Grundy P, Polychronakos C. Aberrant imprinting of the insulin-like growth factor II receptor gene in Wilms' tumor. Oncogene 1997; 14(9): 1041-1046.

[87] Ribarska T, Ingenwerth M, Goering W, Engers R, Schulz WA. Epigenetic inactivation of the placentally imprinted tumor suppressor gene TFPI2 in prostate carcinoma. Cancer Genomics & Proteomics 2010; 7(2): 51-60.

[88] Nakano S, Murakami K, Meguro M, Soejima H, Higashimoto K, Urano T, Kugoh H, Mukai T, Ikeguchi M, Oshimura M. Expression profile of LIT1/KCNQ1OT1 and epigenetic status at the KvDMR1 in colorectal cancers. Cancer Science 2006; 97(11): 1147-1154.

[89] Lu Y, Lu P, Zhu Z, Xu H, Zhu X. Loss of imprinting of insulin-like growth factor 2 is associated with increased risk of lymph node metastasis and gastric corpus cancer. Journal of Experimental & Clinical Cancer Research 2009; 28: 125.

[90] Poirier K, Chalas C, Tissier F, Couvert P, Mallet V, Carrié A, Marchio A, Sarli D, Gicquel C, Chaussade S, Beljord C, Chelly J, Kerjean A, Terris B. Loss of parental-specific methylation at the IGF2 locus in human hepatocellular carcinoma. The Journal of Pathology 2003; 201(3): 473-479.

[91] Dejeux E, Olaso R, Dousset B, Audebourg A, Gut IG, Terris B, Tost J. Hypermethylation of the IGF2 differentially methylated region 2 is a specific event in insulinomas

leading to loss-of-imprinting and overexpression. Endocrine-Related Cancer 2009; 16(3): 939-952.

[92] Vu TH, Chuyen NV, Li T, Hoffman AR. Loss of imprinting of IGF2 sense and antisense transcripts in Wilms' tumor. Cancer Research 2003; 63(8): 1900-1905.

[93] Elkin M, Shevelev A, Schulze E, Tykocinsky M, Cooper M, Ariel I, Pode D, Kopf E, de Groot N, Hochberg A. The expression of the imprinted *H19* and *IGF-2* genes in human bladder carcinoma. FEBS Letters 1995; 374: 57-61.

[94] Xin Z, Soejima H, Higashimoto K, Yatsuki H, Zhu X, Satoh Y, Masaki Z, Kaneko Y, Jinno Y, Fukuzawa R, Hata J, Mukai T. A novel imprinted gene, KCNQ1DN, within the WT2 critical region of human chromosome 11p15.5 and its reduced expression in Wilms' tumors. The Journal of Biological Chemistry 2000; 128(5): 847-853.

[95] Gallagher E, Mc Goldrick A, Chung WY, Mc Cormack O, Harrison M, Kerin M, Dervan PA, Mc Cann A. Gain of imprinting of SLC22A18 sense and antisense transcripts in human breast cancer. Genomics 2006; 88(1): 12-17.

[96] Dallosso AR, Hancock AL, Malik S, Salpekar A, King-Underwood L, Pritchard-Jones K, Peters J, Moorwood K, Ward A, Malik KT, Brown KW. Alternately spliced WT1 antisense transcripts interact with WT1 sense RNA and show epigenetic and splicing defects in cancer. RNA 2007; 13(12): 2287-2299.

[97] Jiang X, Yu Y, Yang HW, Agar NY, Frado L, Johnson MD. The imprinted gene PEG3 inhibits Wnt signaling and regulates glioma growth. The Journal of Biological Chemistry 2010; 285(11): 8472-8480.

[98] Otsuka S, Maegawa S, Takamura A, Kamitani H, Watanabe T, Oshimura M, Nanba E. Aberrant promoter methylation and expression of the imprinted PEG3 gene in glioma. Proceedings of the Japan Academy - Series B: Physical & Biological Sciences 2009; 85(4): 157-165.

[99] Feng W, Marquez RT, Lu Z, Liu J, Lu KH, Issa JP, Fishman DM, Yu Y, Bast RC Jr. Imprinted tumor suppressor genes ARHI and PEG3 are the most frequently down-regulated in human ovarian cancers by loss of heterozygosity and promoter methylation. Cancer 2008; 112(7): 1489-1502.

[100] Tian F, Tang Z, Song G, Pan Y, He B, Bao Q, Wang S. Loss of imprinting of IGF2 correlates with hypomethylation of the H19 differentially methylated region in the tumor tissue of colorectal cancer patients. Molecular Medicine Reports 2012; 5(6): 1536-1540.

[101] Dammann RH, Kirsch S, Schagdarsurengin U, Dansranjavin T, Gradhand E, Schmitt WD, Hauptmann S. Frequent aberrant methylation of the imprinted IGF2/H19 locus and LINE1 hypomethylation in ovarian carcinoma. International Journal of Oncology 2010; 36(1): 171-179.

[102] Honda S, Arai Y, Haruta M, Sasaki F, Ohira M, Yamaoka H, Horie H, Nakagawara A, Hiyama E, Todo S, Kaneko Y. Loss of imprinting of IGF2 correlates with hyperme-

thylation of the H19 differentially methylated region in hepatoblastoma. British Journal of Cancer 2008; 99(11): 1891-1899.

[103] Grbesa I, Marinkovic M, Ivkic M, Kruslin B, Novak-Kujundzic R, Pegan B, Bogdanovic O, Bedekovic V, Gall-Troselj K. Loss of imprinting of IGF2 and H19, loss of heterozygosity of IGF2R and CTCF, and Helicobacter pylori infection in laryngeal squamous cell carcinoma. Journal of Molecular Medicine 2008; 86(9): 1057-1066.

[104] Stier S, Neuhaus T, Albers P, Wernert N, Grünewald E, Forkert R, Vetter H, Ko Y. Loss of imprinting of the insulin-like growth factor 2 and the H19 gene in testicular seminomas detected by real-time PCR approach. Archives of Toxicology 2006; 80(10): 713-718.

[105] Paradowska A, Fenic I, Konrad L, Sturm K, Wagenlehner F, Weidner W, Steger K. Aberrant epigenetic modifications in the CTCF binding domain of the IGF2/H19 gene in prostate cancer compared with benign prostate hyperplasia. International Journal of Oncology 2009; 35(1): 87-96.

[106] el-Naggar AK, Lai S, Tucker SA, Clayman GL, Goepfert H, Hong WK, Huff V. Frequent loss of imprinting at the IGF2 and H19 genes in head and neck squamous carcinoma. Oncogene 1999 25; 18(50): 7063-7069.

[107] Ulaner GA, Vu TH, Li T, Hu JF, Yao XM, Yang Y, Gorlick R, Meyers P, Healey J, Ladanyi M, Hoffman AR. Loss of imprinting of IGF2 and H19 in osteosarcoma is accompanied by reciprocal methylation changes of a CTCF-binding site. Human Molecular Genetics 2003; 12(5):535-549.

[108] Takai D, Gonzales FA, Tsai YC, Thayer MJ, Jones PA. Large scale mapping of methylcytosines in CTCF-binding sites in the human *H19* promoter and aberrant hypomethylation in human bladder cancer. Human Molecular Genetics 2001; 10(23): 2619-2626.

[109] Enokida H, Nakagawa M. Epigenetics in bladder cancer. International Journal of Clinical Oncology 2008; 13: 298–307.

[110] Tanaka MF, Sonpavde G. Diagnosis and management of urothelial carcinoma of then bladder. Postgraduate Medicine 2011; 123(3): 43-55.

[111] Han H, Wolff EM, Liang G. Epigenetic alterations in bladder cancer and their potential clinical implications. Advances in Urology 2012; 2012:546917.

[112] Kim WJ, Bae SC. Molecular biomarkers in urothelial bladder cancer. Cancer Science 2008; 99(4): 646-652.

[113] Proctor I, Stoeber K, Williams GH. Biomarkers in bladder cancer. Histopathology 2010; 57(1): 1-13.

[114] Oudejans CB, Mulders J, Lachmeijer AM, van Dijk M, Könst AA, Westerman BA, van Wijk IJ, Leegwater PA, Kato HD, Matsuda T, Wake N, Dekker GA, Pals G, ten Kate LP, Blankenstein MA. The parent-of-origin effect of 10q22 in pre-eclamptic females

coincides with two regions clustered for genes with down-regulated expression in androgenetic placentas. Molecular Human Reproduction 2004; 10(8): 589-598.

[115] van Dijk M, Mulders J, Könst A, Janssens B, van Roy F, Blankenstein M, Oudejans C. Differential down-regulation of alphaT-catenin expression in placenta: trophoblast cell type-dependent imprinting of the CTNNA3 gene. Gene Expression Patterns 2004; 5(1): 61-65.

[116] Meehan M, Melvin A, Gallagher E, Smith J, McGoldrick A, Moss C, Goossens S, Harrison M, Kay E, Fitzpatrick J, Dervan P, Mc Cann A.Alpha-T-catenin (CTNNA3) displays tumour specific monoallelic expression in urothelial carcinoma of the bladder. Genes, Chromosomes and Cancer 2007; 46(6): 587-593.

[117] Lee MH, Yang HY. Negative regulators of cyclin-dependent kinases and their roles in cancers. Cellular and Molecular Life Sciences 2001; 58(12-13): 1907-1922.

[118] Bozdoğan O, Atasoy P, Batislam E, Başar MM, Başar H. Significance of p57(Kip2) down-regulation in oncogenesis of bladder carcinoma: an immunohistochemical study. Tumori 2008; 94(4): 556-562.

[119] Oya M, Schulz WA. Decreased expression of p57(KIP2) mRNA in human bladder cancer. British Journal of Cancer 2000; 83(5): 626-631.

[120] Hao Y, Cernshaw T, Moulton T, Newcomb E, Tycko B. Tumor suppressor activity of *H19* RNA. Nature 1993; 365: 764-767.

[121] Ariel I, Lustig O, Schneider T, Pizov G, Sappir M, de Groot N, Hochberg A. The imprinted *H19* gene as a tumor marker in bladder carcinoma. Urology 1995; 45: 335-338.

[122] Ayesh S, Matouk I, Schneider T, Ohana P, Laster M, Al Sharef W, De-Groot N, Hochberg A. Possible physiological role of *H19* RNA. Molecular Carcinogenesis 2002; 35: 63-74.

[123] Cai X, Cullen BR. The imprinted *H19* noncoding RNA is a primary microRNA precursor. RNA 2007; 13: 313-316.

[124] Cooper MJ, Fischer M, Komitowski D, Shevelev A, Schulze E, Ariel I, Tykocinski ML, Miron S, Ilan J, de Groot N, Hochberg A. Developmentally imprinted genes as markers for bladder tumor progression. The Journal of Urology 1996; 255: 2120-2127.

[125] Byun HM, Wong HL, Birnstein EA, Wolff EM, Liang G, Yang AS. Examination of *IGF2* and *H19* Loss of Imprinting in Bladder Cancer. Cancer Research 2007; 67: 10753-10758.

[126] McConkey DJ, Lee S, Choi W, Tran M, Majewski T, Lee S, Siefker-Radtke A, Dinney C, Czerniak B. Molecular genetics of bladder cancer: Emerging mechanisms of tumor initiation and progression. Urologic Oncology 2010; 28(4): 429-440.

[127] Samani AA, Yakar S, LeRoith D, Brodt P. The role of the IGF system in cancer growth and metastasis: overview and recent insights. Endocrine Reviews 2007; 28(1): 20-47.

[128] Gallagher EM, O'Shea DM, Fitzpatrick P, Harrison M, Gilmartin B, Watson JA, Clarke T, Leonard MO, McGoldrick A, Meehan M, Watson C, Furlong F, O'Kelly P, Fitzpatrick JM, Dervan PA, O'Grady A, Kay EW, McCann A. Recurrence of urothelial carcinoma of the bladder: a role for insulin-like growth factor-II loss of imprinting and cytoplasmic E-cadherin immunolocalization. Clinical Cancer Research 2008; 14(21): 6829-6838.

[129] Chen LM, Verity NJ, Chai KX. Loss of prostasin (PRSS8) in human bladder transitional cell carcinoma cell lines is associated with epithelial-mesenchymal transition (EMT). BMC Cancer 2009; 9: 377.

[130] Boyer B, Vallés AM, Edme N. Induction and regulation of epithelial-mesenchymal transitions. Biochemical Pharmacology 2000; 60(8): 1091-1099.

[131] Morali OG, Delmas V, Moore R, Jeanney C, Thiery JP, Larue L IGF-II induces rapid beta-catenin relocation to the nucleus during epithelium to mesenchyme transition. Oncogene 2001; 20(36): 4942-4950.

[132] Elkin M, Ayesh S, Schneider T, de Groot N, Hochberg A, Ariel I. The dynamics of the imprinted *H19* gene expression in the mouse model of bladder carcinoma induced by N-butyl-N-(4-hydroxybutyl)nitrosamine. Carcinogenesis 1998; 19(12): 2095-2099.

[133] Ohana P, Bibi O, Matouk I, Levy C, Birman T, Ariel I, Schneider T, Ayesh S, Giladi H, Laster M, de Groot N, Hochberg A. Use of *H19* regulatory sequences for targeted gene therapy in cancer. International Journal of Cancer 2002; 98(5): 645-650.

[134] Amit D, Hochberg A. Development of targeted therapy for bladder cancer mediated by a double promoter plasmid expressing diphtheria toxin under the control of *H19* and *IGF2*-P4 regulatory sequences. Journal of Translational Medicine 2010; 8:134.

[135] Moreira JM, Ohlsson G, Gromov P, Simon R, Sauter G, Celis JE, Gromova I. Bladder cancer-associated protein, a potential prognostic biomarker in human bladder cancer. Molecular & Cellular Proteomics 2010; 9(1): 161-177.

[136] Gromova I, Gromov P, Celis JE. bc10: A novel human bladder cancer-associated protein with a conserved genomic structure downregulated in invasive cancer. International Journal of Cancer 2002; 98(4): 539-546.

[137] Rae FK, Stephenson SA, Nicol DL, Clements JA. Novel association of a diverse range of genes with renal cell carcinoma as identified by differential display. International Journal of Cancer 2000; 88(5): 726-732.

[138] Zuo Z, Zhao M, Liu J, Gao G, Wu X. Functional analysis of bladder cancer-related protein gene: a putative cervical cancer tumor suppressor gene in cervical carcinoma. Tumour Biology 2006; 27(4): 221-226.

[139] Daino K, Ugolin N, Altmeyer-Morel S, Guilly MN, Chevillard S. Gene expression profiling of alpha-radiation-induced rat osteosarcomas: identification of dysregulat-

ed genes involved in radiation-induced tumorigenesis of bone. International Journal of Cancer 2009; 125(3): 612-620.

[140] Fan DG, Zhao F, Ding Y, Wu MM, Fan QY, Shimizu K, Dohjima T, Nozawa S, Wakahara K, Ohno T, Guo YS, Ma BA, Jiang JL. *BLCAP* induces apoptosis in human Ewing's sarcoma cells. Experimental Biology and Medicine 2011; 236(9): 1030-1035.

[141] Evans HK, Wylie AA, Murphy SK, Jirtle RL. The neuronatin gene resides in a "microimprinted" domain on human chromosome 20q11.2. Genomics 2001; 77(1-2): 99-104.

[142] Schulz R, McCole RB, Woodfine K, Wood AJ, Chahal M, Monk D, Moore GE, Oakey RJ. Transcript- and tissue-specific imprinting of a tumour suppressor gene. Human and Molecular Genetics 2009; 18(1): 118-127.

[143] Kanber D, Berulava T, Ammerpohl O, Mitter D, Richter J, Siebert R, Horsthemke B, Lohmann D, Buiting K. The human retinoblastoma gene is imprinted. PLoS Genetics 2009; 5(12):e1000790.

[144] Buiting K, Kanber D, Horsthemke B, Lohmann D. Imprinting of *RB1* (the new kid on the block). Briefings in Functional Genomics 2010; 9(4): 347-353.

[145] Nakabayashi K, Trujillo AM, Tayama C, Camprubi C, Yoshida W, Lapunzina P, Sanchez A, Soejima H, Aburatani H, Nagae G, Ogata T, Hata K, Monk D. Methylation screening of reciprocal genome-wide UPDs identifies novel human-specific imprinted genes. Human Molecular Genetics 2011; 20(16): 3188-3197.

[146] Chinnam M, Goodrich DW. *RB1*, development, and cancer. Current Topics in Developmental Biology 2011; 94: 129-169.

[147] Quentin T, Henke C, Korabiowska M, Schlott T, Zimmerman B, Kunze E. Altered mRNA expression of the Rb and p16 tumor suppressor genes and of CDK4 in transitional cell carcinomas of the urinary bladder associated with tumor progression. Anticancer Research 2004; 24(2B): 1011-1023.

[148] Abdulamir AS, Hafidh RR, Kadhim HS, Abubakar F. Tumor markers of bladder cancer: the schistosomal bladder tumors versus non-schistosomal bladder tumors. Journal of Experimental & Clinical Cancer Research 2009; 28: 27.

[149] Dulaimi E, Uzzo RG, Greenberg RE, Al-Saleem T, Cairns P. Detection of bladder cancer in urine by a tumor suppressor gene hypermethylation panel. Clinical Cancer Research 2004; 10(6): 1887-1893.

[150] Agundez M, Grau L, Palou J, Algaba F, Villavicencio H, Sanchez-Carbayo M. Evaluation of the methylation status of tumour suppressor genes for predicting bacillus Calmette-Guérin response in patients with T1G3 high-risk bladder tumours. European Urology 2011; 60(1): 131-140.

[151] Kaghad M, Bonnet H, Yang A, Creancier L, Biscan JC, Valent A, Minty A, Chalon P, Lelias JM, Dumont X, Ferrara P, McKeon F, Caput D. Monoallelically expressed gene

related to p53 at 1p36, a region frequently deleted in neuroblastoma and other human cancers. Cell 1997; 90(4): 809-819.

[152] Judson H, van Roy N, Strain L, Vandesompele J, Van Gele M, Speleman F, Bonthron DT. Structure and mutation analysis of the gene encoding DNA fragmentation factor 40 (caspase-activated nuclease), a candidate neuroblastoma tumour suppressor gene. Human Genetics 2000; 106(4): 406-413.

[153] Stiewe T, Pützer BM. Role of p73 in malignancy: tumor suppressor or oncogene? Cell Death and Differentiation 20029(3): 237-245.

[154] Chen CL, Ip SM, Cheng D, Wong LC, Ngan HY. P73 gene expression in ovarian cancer tissues and cell lines. Clinical Cancer Research 2000; 6(10): 3910-3915.

[155] Zaika AI, Kovalev S, Marchenko ND, Moll UM. Overexpression of the wild type p73 gene in breast cancer tissues and cell lines. Cancer Research 1999; 59(13): 3257-3263.

[156] Kang MJ, Park BJ, Byun DS, Park JI, Kim HJ, Park JH, Chi SG. Loss of imprinting and elevated expression of wild-type p73 in human gastric adenocarcinoma. Clinical Cancer Research 2000; 6(5): 1767-1771.

[157] Chi SG, Chang SG, Lee SJ, Lee CH, Kim JI, Park JH. Elevated and biallelic expression of p73 is associated withprogression of human bladder cancer. Cancer Research 1999; 59(12): 2791-2793.

[158] Yokomizo A, Mai M, Tindall DJ, Cheng L, Bostwick DG, Naito S, Smith DI, Liu W. Overexpression of the wild type p73 gene in human bladder cancer. Oncogene 1999; 18(8): 1629-1633.

[159] Jelinic P, Shaw P. Loss of imprinting and cancer. The Journal of Pathology 2007; 211(3): 261-268.

Chapter 4

The Changing Incidence of Carcinoma In-Situ of the Bladder Worldwide

Weranja Ranasinghe and Raj Persad

Additional information is available at the end of the chapter

http://dx.doi.org/10.5772/53929

1. Introduction

Bladder carcinoma is the sixth most common cancer worldwide with increasing health-care burden and treatment costs [1-3]. The majority (70%) of bladder cancers are superficial tumours which require close observation with repeat cystocopy, timely resection and long term follow-up. Of these superficial bladder cancers, 10% are carcinoma in situ [4].

Originally described by Melicow in 1952 [5], carcinoma in situ(CIS) of the bladder is defined as a flat (e.g. non-papillary) high-grade non-invasive urothelial carcinoma (transitional cell carcinoma) [6]. An important distinction is that CIS of the urinary bladder, unlike testicular and prostatic CIS, 'in situ' disease is not a precursor to malignancy but is a malignant entity in its own right [6, 7] which has over 50% five-year progression rate in untreated disease and higher recurrence rates [8, 9].

CIS is characterised by a flat 'red velvet' lesion which is usually multifocal and predominantly found in the trigone region, peri ureteral areas and the bladder neck with frequent involvement of the posterior and lateral walls [10]. Extra-vesical CIS is frequently found in the ureters and prostatic urethra.

The microscopic features of CIS (Figure 1) are nuclear anaplasia (identical to that of high grade urothelial carcinoma) containing large irregular, hyperchromic nuclei (3 to 5 times the size of a lymphocyte) and frequent mitotic activity and usually observed in part of or the entire thickness of epithelium in the mid to upper urinary tract [11, 12]. Immunohistologically, these cells also stain diffusely positive for CK20 and expresses p53 [11].

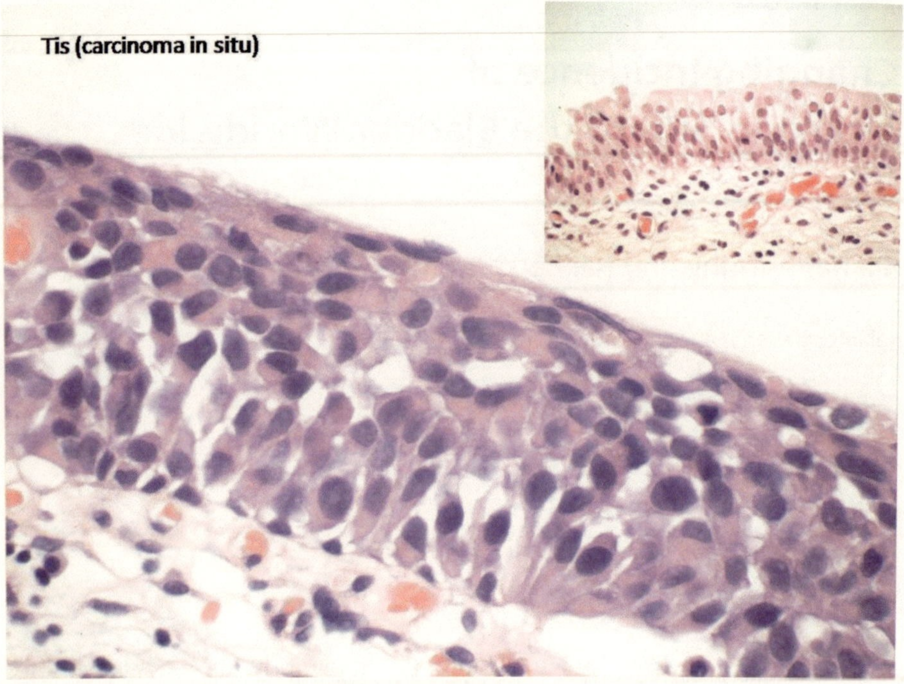

Figure 1. This figure demonstrates the histological features of CIS.

2. Classification of CIS

CIS was previously categorised under the broad term 'moderate/severe dysplasia or marked atypia' [11] where the grade was determined by the degree/severity of dysplasia. However, the grading of bladder cancers has been subject to much controversy and a more comprehensive classification system was published by the World Health Organisation and the International Society of Urological Pathology (WHO/ISUP) in 1998 [13]. The current WHO/ISUP classification states that *'by definition, all CIS are high-grade lesions. CIS should not be sub classified by grade, despite the spectrum of pleomorphism seen within this entity'* [11].

The TNM bladder cancer staging system also acknowledges CIS as a separate entity (Tis); however, it is classified along with the low grade Ta and T1 tumours in bladder tumours.

Different classifications have been suggested in order to stratify risk and prognosis of CIS. One of the methods used to determine the prognosis of CIS was by the presence of symptoms, number of sites of involved (multifocal vs. unifocal) and concurrent CIS with papillary tumours. However these features have not been completely validated [7].

A currently used classification of CIS [7, 10, 14] is:

- Primary (isolated lesion in the bladder urothelium with no previous or concurrent papillary tumours).
- Secondary (CIS detected during the follow-up of patients with a previous papillary tumour).
- Concurrent (CIS in the presence of papillary tumours).

Primary CIS has a worse outcome with higher rates of progression to muscle invasive disease resulting in a higher rates of cystectomy; but is shown to respond better to BCG therapy compared to secondary CIS [15]. A further study confirmed the higher rates of progression to muscle invasive disease in primary CIS, while concurrent CIS was shown to have the worst survival rates [16]. This highlights the importance of differentiating between the types of CIS in determining the prognosis and also identifying primary CIS early.

3. Incidence

Although increases in the incidences of bladder cancer in the USA, Japan and European countries have been observed in recent decades [1, 2], the incidence of primary CIS remains largely unknown. This is mainly due to bladder CIS being classified as a 'premalignant condition' with other 'in situ' diseases and therefore is a non-reportable condition in many countries. An excellent example is that CIS and pTa bladder carcinomas are registered alongside malignant disease in North America but not the UK [17]. However, more cancer registries are recommended to include CIS as a reportable malignancy, as these 'unreported' increasing incidences can sometimes go unnoticed [18].

The literature suggests that between 5-10% of bladder carcinomas are CIS but this could be as high as 19 % [14]. Our analysis of the Surveillance Epidemiology and End Result (SEER) database [19] revealed an incidence of 14 per 100,000 persons where CIS was the primary coded tumour from 1973 -2009. The incidence of CIS in males and females in the US were 24.9 and 6.2 per 100,000, respectively. In comparison the incidence of malignant bladder cancer was 27 per 100,000 in males and 6.8 per 100,000 in females, for the same duration. In addition, there was a 28% increase in the overall incidence of CIS from 1975, with 27% and 20% seen in males and females respectively. On a Joinpoint regression analysis [20], there was a significant 0.3% annual percentage increase in males since 1990, but not in females. It should be noted that these CIS rates could also include secondary and concurrent CIS.

In Australia the incidence of primary CIS was 20.9 per 100,000 and 6.5 per 100,000 in males and females >50 years respectively, with an 11% and 14% annual increase seen from 2001 onwards [18].

There could be significant variation in the reported incidence of CIS in cancer registry data due to a variety of factors such as inter- observer variability in categorisation of the tumour, coding differences and increasing awareness of CIS. Similarly, re-resection of the tumours can upstage an initial diagnosis of a tumour. In addition, being an unreported malignancy, there is significant emphasis being placed on the hospital coding to determine the incidence of CIS and it can also be difficult to determine if the diagnoses coded as CIS are histologically proven post biopsy or if they are based on cytology alone. Furthermore, increasing awareness with higher screening or investigation rates could play an important role in increased number of diagnoses of CIS.

These factors provide some limitations for determining the actual incidence of CIS. However, importance of recording the trends of CIS is essential and may help observe for any increases in incidence and initiate awareness and early intervention.

4. Risk factors

4.1. Gender and age

Male gender is a well documented risk factor in bladder cancer with males having a 4.1 fold increase compared to females [1]. As with bladder carcinoma, male gender tends to have a higher preponderance for CIS than females with 3.1-7 times risk of developing CIS [18, 21, 22].

Increasing age is also a risk factor for bladder cancer. The highest incidences of bladder cancer are seen in the >50 year olds [23] while the mean incidence for patients with CIS also occurs between the ages of 65-73 years [21, 22].

4.2. Smoking

Smoking is one of the major risk factors for bladder cancer. Smoking increases the risk of bladder cancer by 2- 6 fold which is augmented by increasing duration and frequency of smoking, while cessation of smoking decreases this risk [2]. The effects of long term smoking are found to carry similar risks for developing bladder cancer in both sexes [24].

Although not many studies have focussed exclusively on the relationship of CIS and smoking, there is evidence to establish smoking as a risk factor for CIS. In a study which focussed only on CIS, the 72% of patients who presented with CIS were either former or current smokers [15]. In a another study of all superficial bladder tumours, which included CIS, showed that those who continued to smoke after the diagnosis of the tumour, had worse bladder cancer related outcomes with a shorter time to disease recurrence, while ex-smokers tended to present with a tumour at a later age [25]. However, the link between smoking and failure of BCG therapy bladder tumours is not very clear [26].

Despite the strong links between smoking and bladder cancer, smoking can only partially account for the incidence of bladder cancer suggesting that other risk factors also contribute to the risks [27].

4.3. Schitosomiasis infection

Schistosoma haematobium or Bilharzia is a known pathogen for causing bladder cancer in the prevalent areas and accounts for about 3% of the world bladder cancer [2]. Infection with schistosomiasis increases the risk of bladder cancer by 5 fold and accounts for majority of the incidence squamous cell bladder cancers [2]. However, CIS has been also seen in patients with Schistosomial infection where the pathogenesis is thought to be linked to chromosomal loss [28].

4.4. Occupational carcinogens

There is a well established link between occupational carcinogen and bladder cancer with an estimated 20- 27% of bladder cancers attributed to occupational exposures. The main carcinogens associated with industrial occupational risk are aromatic amines (beta-naphthylamine, 4-aminobiphenyl and benzidine) which are used widely as intermediary compounds in the textile and rubber industries. The risk of occupational bladder cancer is dependent not only on the intensity and characteristics of the workplace exposures, but also on individual susceptibility to these cancers [29]. Similar to bladder carcinoma, CISs also develops in patients exposed to these carcinogens [30] where mutations of the p53 gene is thought to initiate the disease process [31]

4.5. Genes

Polymorphisms in the genes, NAT2 and GSTM1 are the main genetic modulations implicated in the bladder cancer. NAT 2 encodes the N-acetyltransferase 2 enzyme responsible for detoxification of aromatic amines by N-acetylation or activation by O-acetylation, while GSTM1 encodes the glutathione S-transferase M1 enzyme responsible for detoxification of carcinogens such as polycyclic aromatic hydrocarbons and reactive oxygen species. [32] In CIS however, the genetic mutations are different and characterized by loss-of-function of the tumour suppressor genes, such as p53, RB, and PTEN [33]. These genetic changes are discussed in detail in another chapter.

4.6. Diet

Dietary factors are also shown to be linked to bladder cancer. Fruit and vegetative intake correspond inversely with the risk of bladder cancer while there is evidence to show that Vitamin B and yellow orange vegetables (in individuals with the presence of GSTM1) may also reduce the risk of bladder cancer [32]. However, to our knowledge, there are no specific studies looking at the dietary risks and CIS.

5. Presentation

Presentation of primary CIS of the bladder can be very variable (Table 1). Majority of the patients with primary CIS present with only non-specific irritative bladder symptoms such as dysuria, frequency, urgency or nocturia [15] [21, 22, 34]. Furthermore up to 22- 26% of patients are asymptomatic and less commonly may present with suprapubic fullness or pain, back or flank discomfort, lower abdominal pain, or pelvic-perineal pain [15, 21, 22]. In contrast with bladder cancer, fewer than 45% of the patients have macroscopic or microscopic haematuria in primary disease [22], highlighting the difficulty in diagnosing this condition. In contrast, the patients with secondary or concomitant CIS tend to present with gross haematuria, possibly due to the presence of a papillary tumour [15].

Symptom	% with symptom	
	Primary CIS	Secondary/concomitant CIS
Irritative	28.5(15)	9.8(15)
Asymptomatic	22(15)- 26(22)	21(15)
Macroscopic haematuria	31.2(15)	50.6(15)

Table 1. The percentage of patients presenting with various symptoms of primary and secondary/concomitant CIS.

6. Diagnostic workup

6.1. Biopsy of the red velvet lesion

The diagnosis of CIS can be challenging task due to the flat nature of the lesion, where the mucosa containing the lesion could be unremarkable or simply an erosion [21]. Therefore, biopsy of the lesion is the current advocated method for diagnosis of CIS of the bladder. However, even the characteristic 'red velvety patch' of CIS could be non-specific [21] and the specificity could be as low as 8% [35]. Thus it is recommended that the biopsies of even the normal mucosa are taken in high risk patient or in the presence of positive cytology [14, 21].

In addition, a second look transurethral resection (TUR) and bladder mapping biopsies are frequently warranted to reduce under staging, exclude residual disease and concurrent CIS in patients with other bladder tumours [15].

6.2. White light cystoscopy vs. fluorescent light cystoscopy

One of the difficulties during cystoscopy is the visualisation of this flat lesion in the bladder, which could be inconspicuous under normal white light cystoscopy and can be missed resulting in significantly under-reporting. The recent use of fluorescent light cystoscopy using 5-aminolevulinic acid or hexaminolevulinate has been shown to enhance the detection of CIS by more than 30%- 39% [36, 37] and also to reduce tumour recurrence at 1 and 2 years [38]. When using florescent light cystoscopy, both 5-aminolevulinic acid and hexaminolevulinate are shown to be equally effective at detecting CIS [37]. In addition, the use of HAL when resecting tumours is shown to reduce tumour recurrence in CIS and also in multifocal tumours [39]. Despite the benefits of fluorescent light cystoscopy, one of its major drawbacks is the high false positive rates. The European Urology Association guidelines recommendations of the use of fluorescent light cystoscopy due to its high sensitivity [14], but it is not universally used in practice due to availability and cost implications.

6.3. Biomarkers

Biomarkers have been widely used in aiding the detection of CIS. Some of the routinely used biomarkers are urine cytology, UroVysion (fluorescent in-situ hybridization - FISH), immunocytology and Nuclear Matrix Protein (NMP22). Of these, urine cytology is the most frequently used in detecting CIS due to its high sensitivity. However the specificity of cytology, FISH and immunocytology are all below 30% limiting the diagnostic accuracy of CIS [40]. Even, NMP22 which has the highest specificity for CIS, is only 43% [40] (Table 2).

Modality	Percentage CIS detected
Biopsy of 'red mucosa'	8-78%(44), (35)
Florescent light cystocopy (using 5-aminolevulinic acid or hexaminolevulinic acid)	92.4%(45).
White light cystoscopy	60.5%(45)
Urine Cytology	90% - 92.3(6, 40)
UroVysion (fluorescent in-situ hybridization - FISH)	83.6(40)
Immune-cytology µCyt	81.3(40)
NMP22	79.1(40)
Combination of FISH+ CYT	85.3(40)

Table 2. The percentage of CIS detected by each modality of testing.

Therefore to optimise the accuracy of diagnosis, it is recommended that these biomarkers should be used in conjunction with each other rather than on their own [21]. The use of cytology and NMP22 together increase the specificity 55% and using all 4 modalities increase the sensitivity to 65% [40]. However, due to lower sensitivities of some of these tests, the overall sensitivity decreases as more tests are combined [40]. Therefore an optimum balance must be used to obtain the best sensitivity and specificity values in diagnosis of CIS.

Another very useful role of biomarkers is to predict response to treatment. A number of biomarkers, urine markers and genetic markers have been evaluated to predict which tumours will fail BCG therapy [41]. Interleukin -2 is shown to be promising in in identifying the tumours which will not respond to BCG therapy. However, currently none of the other markers have large studies or long term validation to predict treatment failure prior to starting BCG [41].

6.4. Screening for CIS

The usefulness of biomarkers as screening tools in detection of CIS is suboptimal. A study which screened a group of 183 smokers using a variety of screening tools, showed the true positive rates for detection of malignant tumours were only 50% for Dipstick, 6% for BladderChek, 37% for cytology and 61% for UroVysion (FISH) [42]. The 2 patients with CIS, had negative results for urine dipstick and cytology but were positive for UroVysion [42]. However, another study showed low cost effectiveness of the use of Uro Vysion as a screening tool, due to its high costs [43]. Thus screening for CIS may not be economically viable.

7. Treatment

Studies have demonstrated that the untreated natural history of CIS has a 50% progression rate to malignant disease at 5 years and even with optimal treatment, progression and recurrence rates are both high [8, 9].

7.1. Tumour resection

Transurethral resection (TUR) is essential in providing histological tissue and reducing the tumour load. When the muscularis mucosa is involved, a re-resection is usually necessary. Despite this, in treatment of CIS, solitary TUR is shown to be inferior compared to TUR when used in conjunction with BCG, with the latter having increased the 10 year progression free survival (71% vs. 50%) [46].

7.2. Intravesical Chemotherapy/Immunotherapy

Intravesical instillation of a chemotherapeutic/immunotherapeutic agent is the mainstay treatment for CIS. A number of agents such as Bacille Calmette-Guerin (BCG), mitomycin C, epirubicin, doxorubicin and adriamycin have been trialed. In comparison trails between these agent, BCG is shown to be superior to other chemotherapeutic agents with higher complete response rates (68% vs. 49%) and higher disease free rates (51% vs. 27%) [14]. Furthermore, the use of BCG with maintenance therapy was also superior to mitomycin C [47].

Despite the advantages of BCG therapy, studies have demonstrated that 20% to 40% fail to respond and progress [41]. In addition, up to 90% of patients experience side effects such as local cystitis symptoms such dysuria, frequency alteration, and occasional haematuria resulting a number of patients not completing the treatment schedule [41].

7.3. Radio therapy

Radiotherapy is a is also used as a treatment modality in bladder carcinoma, where radiotherapy is shown to complete local regression of muscle-invasive bladder cancer in upto 73% of patients [48]. However radiotherapy has been shown to be ineffective against CIS of the bladder. In CIS patients treated with EBRT have demonstrated persistent CIS after treatment and was shown to be inferior to radical cystectomy [49, 50]. Furthermore in patients with concomitant CIS treated with radiotherapy, the presence of CIS carried a worse prognosis [51].

7.4. Cystectomy

Cystectomy is an important option in treating CIS of the bladder due to its high cure rates in high risk patients [52] and is advocated in high risk patients. This is especially useful in patients who do not respond to BCG, where early cystectomy is shown to improve long term survival [53]. However, studies have shown that the presence of CIS to be an independent risk factor for upper tract recurrence in patients who undergo cystectomy [54]. In patients with prostatic urethral involvement, immediate or delayed urethrectomy is advocated [55].

7.5. Photodynamic therapy

Photodynamic therapy works by light of a specific wavelength that is absorbed by a chemical photosynthesizer, which then transfers this energy to breakdown oxygen molecules into highly reactive intermediates [56]. An advantage of photodynamic therapy is that the whole bladder mucosa can be treated without having to localise multifocal superficial bladder tumours and occult CIS. A number of photo synthesizers have been used such as Hematoporphyrin derivatives and 5-aminolevulinic Acid (ALA). Photodynamic therapy has been shown to be very promising results in treating CIS, and may provide an alternative treatment for resistance disease [56].

7.6. Treatment for Non-intravesical CIS of the bladder

Extra vesical CIS of the bladder is seen most frequently in the ureters and in the prostatic urethra. In upper tract CIS, BCG therapy is shown to be very effective [57] and the long term data is seen to be as effective as nephroureteroctomy [58]. However, patients who undergo radical nephrectomy and have upper tract concomitant CIS have higher rates of recurrence and poorer cancer specific survival [59].

BCG therapy is also effective in patients with CIS of the prostatic urethra and transurethral resection is thought to have no added advantage [60] However, presence of CIS of the prostatic urethra carries a poorer prognosis and in primary high grade bladder cancers treated with BCG, it is recommended that the prostatic urethra is biopsied as it is a prognostic factor for recurrence, progression of disease and bladder cancer specific mortality [61]. Presence of CIS of the prostatic urethra is also an indication for early cystectomy [62].

7.6.1. Current recommendations for CIS

7.6.1.1. Treatment of primary CIS

The American Urology Association (AUA) guidelines [63] recommend re-resection in high grade disease in the absence of muscularis propria in the specimen as standard treatment followed by an induction course of BCG and maintenance BCG therapy. They suggest that cystectomy also maybe an option in select CIS patients due to high cure rates.

The European Association of Urology (EAU) guidelines [64] state that the BCG installation should be administered for at least 1 year and if the prostatic urethra is involved, TUR of the prostate followed by BCG therapy is recommended for the management of CIS. Unlike the AUA guidelines, cystectectomy is only reserved for BCG failure due to concerns of over-treatment. They suggest 3 monthly follow up cytology with cystoscopy for 2 years and every 6 months thereafter until 5 years followed by annually thereafter. Annual upper tract imaging is also recommended.

7.6.1.2. Treatment of recurrent disease

The AUA guidelines [63] recommend repeat resection in order to aid accurate staging as standard treatment and also recommend cystectomy as an option due to high risk of progression to muscle invasive disease in these patients. They suggest that further intravesical therapy maybe an option.

The EAU [64] guidelines suggest that although further BCG instillation can be beneficial in non-muscle invasive recurrence post chemotherapy, it increase the risk of progression in CIS and they recommend the use of early cystectomy following BCG failure in suitable patients. They further acknowledge that although device assisted chemotherapy instillation and use of concomitant interferon alpha maybe beneficial in select patients, they feel that they are still experimental.

In conclusion, this chapter discusses the incidence, diagnostic difficulty and management of CIS and also the current recommended guidelines.

Acknowledgements

We would like to thank Mr. Salah Al-Buheissi, specialist registrar at the Bristol Royal Infirmary for his input in revision of this manuscript. We would also like to thank Dr. M. Sohail, consultant senior lecturer at the department of cellular and molecular medicine, Severn Deanery for the histology slides.

Author details

Weranja Ranasinghe[1] and Raj Persad[2]

1 Alfred Hospital, Melbourne, Australia

2 University Hospitals Bristol, Bristol, United Kingdom

http://dx.doi.org/10.5772/53929

References

[1] Ferlay J SH, Bray F, Forman D, Mathers C and Parkin DM. GLOBOCAN 2008, Cancer Incidence and Mortality Worldwide: IARC CancerBase No. 10 [Internet]. Lyon, France: International Agency for Research on Cancer; 2010 [cited 2010 July]; Available from: http://globocan.iarc.fr.

[2] Parkin DM. The global burden of urinary bladder cancer. Scand J Urol Nephrol Suppl. 2008(218):12-20. Epub 2008/12/06.

[3] Sievert KD, Amend B, Nagele U, Schilling D, Bedke J, Horstmann M, et al. Economic aspects of bladder cancer: what are the benefits and costs? World J Urol. 2009;27(3): 295-300. Epub 2009/03/10.

[4] Kirkali Z, Chan T, Manoharan M, Algaba F, Busch C, Cheng L, et al. Bladder cancer: epidemiology, staging and grading, and diagnosis. Urology. 2005;66(6 Suppl 1):4-34. Epub 2006/01/10.

[5] Melicow MM, Hollowell JW. Intra-urothelial cancer: carcinoma in situ, Bowen's disease of the urinary system: discussion of thirty cases. J Urol. 1952;68(4):763-72. Epub 1952/10/01.

[6] Witjes JA. Bladder carcinoma in situ in 2003: state of the art. Eur Urol. 2004;45(2): 142-6. Epub 2004/01/22.

[7] Sylvester RJ, van der Meijden A, Witjes JA, Jakse G, Nonomura N, Cheng C, et al. High-grade Ta urothelial carcinoma and carcinoma in situ of the bladder. Urology. 2005;66(6 Suppl 1):90-107. Epub 2006/01/10.

[8] Wolf H, Melsen F, Pedersen SE, Nielsen KT. Natural history of carcinoma in situ of the urinary bladder. Scand J Urol Nephrol Suppl. 1994;157:147-51. Epub 1994/01/01.

[9] Lamm DL. Carcinoma in situ. Urol Clin North Am. 1992;19(3):499-508. Epub 1992/08/01.

[10] Lamm D, Herr H, Jakse G, Kuroda M, Mostofi FK, Okajima E, et al. Updated concepts and treatment of carcinoma in situ. Urol Oncol. 1998;4(4-5):130-8. Epub 1998/07/01.

[11] Epstein JI. Diagnosis and classification of flat, papillary, and invasive urothelial carcinoma: the WHO/ISUP consensus. Int J Surg Pathol. 2010;18(3 Suppl):106S-11S. Epub 2010/05/28.

[12] Humphrey PA. Urothelial carcinoma in situ of the bladder. J Urol. 2012;187(3):1057-8. Epub 2012/01/24.

[13] Pasin E, Josephson DY, Mitra AP, Cote RJ, Stein JP. Superficial bladder cancer: an update on etiology, molecular development, classification, and natural history. Rev Urol. 2008;10(1):31-43. Epub 2008/05/13.

[14] van der Meijden AP, Sylvester R, Oosterlinck W, Solsona E, Boehle A, Lobel B, et al. EAU guidelines on the diagnosis and treatment of urothelial carcinoma in situ. Eur Urol. 2005;48(3):363-71. Epub 2005/07/05.

[15] Chade DC, Shariat SF, Adamy A, Bochner BH, Donat SM, Herr HW, et al. Clinical outcome of primary versus secondary bladder carcinoma in situ. J Urol. 2010;184(2): 464-9. Epub 2010/07/14.

[16] Meijer RP, van Onna IE, Kok ET, Bosch R. The risk profiles of three clinical types of carcinoma in situ of the bladder. BJU Int. 2011;108(6):839-43. Epub 2010/12/21.

[17] Crow P, Ritchie AW. National and international variation in the registration of bladder cancer. BJU Int. 2003;92(6):563-6. Epub 2003/09/27.

[18] Ranasinghe WKB. AJ, Oldmeadow C., Lawrentschuk N., Robertson J., Ranasinghe T., Bolton D., Persad R. Bladder Carcinoma-in-situ in Australia: a rising incidence for an under-reported malignancy. BJUI. 2012.

[19] Surveillance E, and End Results (SEER) Program (www.seer.cancer.gov) SEER*Stat Database: Incidence - SEER 9 Regs Research Data, Nov 2011 Sub, Vintage 2009 Pops (1973-2009) <Katrina/Rita Population Adjustment> - Linked To County Attributes - Total U.S., 1969-2010 Counties, National Cancer Institute, DCCPS, Surveillance Research Program, Surveillance Systems Branch, released April 2012, based on the November 2011 submission.

[20] Joinpoint Regression Program, Version 3.5 - April 2011; Statistical Methodology and Applications Branch and Data Modeling Branch, Surveillance Research Program National Cancer Institute. .

[21] Williamson SR, Montironi R, Lopez-Beltran A, MacLennan GT, Davidson DD, Cheng L. Diagnosis, evaluation and treatment of carcinoma in situ of the urinary bladder: the state of the art. Crit Rev Oncol Hematol. 2010;76(2):112-26. Epub 2010/01/26.

[22] Cheng L, Cheville JC, Neumann RM, Leibovich BC, Egan KS, Spotts BE, et al. Survival of patients with carcinoma in situ of the urinary bladder. Cancer. 1999;85(11): 2469-74. Epub 1999/06/05.

[23] Jemal A, Siegel R, Ward E, Hao Y, Xu J, Murray T, et al. Cancer statistics, 2008. CA Cancer J Clin. 2008;58(2):71-96. Epub 2008/02/22.

[24] Quirk JT, Li Q, Natarajan N, Mettlin CJ, Cummings KM. Cigarette smoking and the risk of bladder cancer in men and women. Tob Induc Dis. 2004;2(3):141-4. Epub 2004/01/01.

[25] Fleshner N, Garland J, Moadel A, Herr H, Ostroff J, Trambert R, et al. Influence of smoking status on the disease-related outcomes of patients with tobacco-associated superficial transitional cell carcinoma of the bladder. Cancer. 1999;86(11):2337-45. Epub 1999/12/11.

[26] Sfakianos JP, Shariat SF, Favaretto RL, Rioja J, Herr HW. Impact of smoking on outcomes after intravesical bacillus Calmette-Guerin therapy for urothelial carcinoma not invading muscle of the bladder. BJU Int. 2011;108(4):526-30. Epub 2010/12/01.

[27] Hemelt M, Yamamoto H, Cheng KK, Zeegers MP. The effect of smoking on the male excess of bladder cancer: a meta-analysis and geographical analyses. Int J Cancer. 2009;124(2):412-9. Epub 2008/09/16.

[28] Khaled HM, Aly MS, Mokhtar N. Chromosomal aberrations in Cis and Ta bilharzial bladder cancer: a theory of pathogenesis. Urol Oncol. 2004;22(6):443-7. Epub 2004/12/22.

[29] Delclos GL, Lerner SP. Occupational risk factors. Scand J Urol Nephrol Suppl. 2008(218):58-63. Epub 2008/12/05.

[30] Crosby JH, Allsbrook WC, Jr., Koss LG, Bales CE, Witherington R, Schulte PA, et al. Cytologic detection of urothelial cancer and other abnormalities in a cohort of workers exposed to aromatic amines. Acta Cytol. 1991;35(3):263-8. Epub 1991/05/01.

[31] Yasunaga Y, Nakanishi H, Naka N, Miki T, Tsujimura T, Itatani H, et al. Alterations of the p53 gene in occupational bladder cancer in workers exposed to aromatic amines. Lab Invest. 1997;77(6):677-84. Epub 1998/01/14.

[32] Garcia-Closas R, Garcia-Closas M, Kogevinas M, Malats N, Silverman D, Serra C, et al. Food, nutrient and heterocyclic amine intake and the risk of bladder cancer. Eur J Cancer. 2007;43(11):1731-40. Epub 2007/06/29.

[33] Castillo-Martin M, Domingo-Domenech J, Karni-Schmidt O, Matos T, Cordon-Cardo C. Molecular pathways of urothelial development and bladder tumorigenesis. Urol Oncol. 2010;28(4):401-8. Epub 2010/07/09.

[34] Hudson MA, Herr HW. Carcinoma in situ of the bladder. J Urol. 1995;153(3 Pt 1): 564-72. Epub 1995/03/01.

[35] Fernando H, Thota SS, Burtt G, Waterfall N, Husain I. Importance of red patches diagnosed in cystoscopy for haematuria and lower urinary tract symptoms. Postgrad Med J. 2007;83(975):62-3. Epub 2007/02/03.

[36] Kausch I, Sommerauer M, Montorsi F, Stenzl A, Jacqmin D, Jichlinski P, et al. Photodynamic diagnosis in non-muscle-invasive bladder cancer: a systematic review and cumulative analysis of prospective studies. Eur Urol. 2010;57(4):595-606. Epub 2009/12/17.

[37] Isfoss BL. The sensitivity of fluorescent-light cystoscopy for the detection of carcinoma in situ (CIS) of the bladder: a meta-analysis with comments on gold standard. BJU Int. 2011;108(11):1703-7. Epub 2011/07/23.

[38] Geavlete B, Multescu R, Georgescu D, Jecu M, Stanescu F, Geavlete P. Treatment changes and long-term recurrence rates after hexaminolevulinate (HAL) fluorescence

cystoscopy: does it really make a difference in patients with non-muscle-invasive bladder cancer (NMIBC)? BJU Int. 2011. Epub 2011/06/30.

[39] Karaolides T, Skolarikos A, Bourdoumis A, Konandreas A, Mygdalis V, Thanos A, et al. Hexaminolevulinate-induced Fluorescence versus White Light During Transurethral Resection of Noninvasive Bladder Tumor: Does It Reduce Recurrences? Urology. 2012;80(2):354-60. Epub 2012/08/04.

[40] Todenhofer T, Hennenlotter J, Aufderklamm S, Kuhs U, Gakis G, Germann M, et al. Individual risk assessment in bladder cancer patients based on a multi-marker panel. J Cancer Res Clin Oncol. 2012. Epub 2012/08/16.

[41] Lima L, Dinis-Ribeiro M, Longatto-Filho A, Santos L. Predictive biomarkers of bacillus calmette-guerin immunotherapy response in bladder cancer: where are we now? Adv Urol. 2012;2012:232609. Epub 2012/08/25.

[42] Steiner H, Bergmeister M, Verdorfer I, Granig T, Mikuz G, Bartsch G, et al. Early results of bladder-cancer screening in a high-risk population of heavy smokers. BJU Int. 2008;102(3):291-6. Epub 2008/03/14.

[43] Ferra S, Denley R, Herr H, Dalbagni G, Jhanwar S, Lin O. Reflex UroVysion testing in suspicious urine cytology cases. Cancer. 2009;117(1):7-14. Epub 2009/04/07.

[44] Swinn MJ, Walker MM, Harbin LJ, Adshead JM, Witherow RO, Vale JA, et al. Biopsy of the red patch at cystoscopy: is it worthwhile? Eur Urol. 2004;45(4):471-4; discussion 4. Epub 2004/03/26.

[45] Isfoss BL. The sensitivity of fluorescent-light cystoscopy for the detection of carcinoma in situ (CIS) of the bladder: a meta-analysis with comments on gold standard. BJU Int. 2011. Epub 2011/07/23.

[46] Zieger K, Jensen KM. Long-term risk of progression of carcinoma in situ of the bladder and impact of bacille Calmette-Guerin immunotherapy on the outcome. Scand J Urol Nephrol. 2011. Epub 2011/07/29.

[47] Malmstrom PU, Sylvester RJ, Crawford DE, Friedrich M, Krege S, Rintala E, et al. An individual patient data meta-analysis of the long-term outcome of randomised studies comparing intravesical mitomycin C versus bacillus Calmette-Guerin for non-muscle-invasive bladder cancer. Eur Urol. 2009;56(2):247-56. Epub 2009/05/05.

[48] Jahnson S, Pedersen J, Westman G. Bladder carcinoma--a 20-year review of radical irradiation therapy. Radiother Oncol. 1991;22(2):111-7. Epub 1991/10/01.

[49] Melamed MR, Voutsa NG, Grabstald H. Natural History and Clinical Behavior of in Situ Carcinoma of the Human Urinary Bladder. Cancer. 1964;17:1533-45. Epub 1964/12/01.

[50] Riddle PR, Chisholm GD, Trott PA, Pugh RC. Flat carcinoma in Situ of bladder. Br J Urol. 1975;47(7):829-33. Epub 1975/01/01.

[51] Chung PW, Bristow RG, Milosevic MF, Yi QL, Jewett MA, Warde PR, et al. Long-term outcome of radiation-based conservation therapy for invasive bladder cancer. Urol Oncol. 2007;25(4):303-9. Epub 2007/07/14.

[52] Hassan JM, Cookson MS, Smith JA, Jr., Johnson DL, Chang SS. Outcomes in patients with pathological carcinoma in situ only disease at radical cystectomy. J Urol. 2004;172(3):882-4. Epub 2004/08/18.

[53] Herr HW, Sogani PC. Does early cystectomy improve the survival of patients with high risk superficial bladder tumors? J Urol. 2001;166(4):1296-9. Epub 2001/09/08.

[54] Takayanagi A, Masumori N, Takahashi A, Takagi Y, Tsukamoto T. Upper urinary tract recurrence after radical cystectomy for bladder cancer: incidence and risk factors. Int J Urol. 2012;19(3):229-33. Epub 2011/11/30.

[55] Ahlering TE, Lieskovsky G, Skinner DG. Indications for urethrectomy in men undergoing single stage radical cystectomy for bladder cancer. J Urol. 1984;131(4):657-9. Epub 1984/04/01.

[56] Shackley DC, Briggs C, Whitehurst C, Betts CD, O'Flynn KJ, Clarke NW, et al. Photodynamic therapy for superficial bladder cancer. Expert Rev Anticancer Ther. 2001;1(4):523-30. Epub 2002/07/13.

[57] Miyake H, Eto H, Hara S, Okada H, Kamidono S, Hara I. Clinical outcome of bacillus Calmette-Guerin perfusion therapy for carcinoma in situ of the upper urinary tract. Int J Urol. 2002;9(12):677-80. Epub 2002/12/21.

[58] Kojima Y, Tozawa K, Kawai N, Sasaki S, Hayashi Y, Kohri K. Long-term outcome of upper urinary tract carcinoma in situ: effectiveness of nephroureterectomy versus bacillus Calmette-Guerin therapy. Int J Urol. 2006;13(4):340-4. Epub 2006/06/01.

[59] Otto W, Shariat SF, Fritsche HM, Gupta A, Matsumoto K, Kassouf W, et al. Concomitant carcinoma in situ as an independent prognostic parameter for recurrence and survival in upper tract urothelial carcinoma: a multicenter analysis of 772 patients. World J Urol. 2011;29(4):487-94. Epub 2011/01/21.

[60] Palou J, Xavier B, Laguna P, Montlleo M, Vicente J. In situ transitional cell carcinoma involvement of prostatic urethra: bacillus Calmette-Guerin therapy without previous transurethral resection of the prostate. Urology. 1996;47(4):482-4. Epub 1996/04/01.

[61] Palou J, Sylvester RJ, Faba OR, Parada R, Pena JA, Algaba F, et al. Female gender and carcinoma in situ in the prostatic urethra are prognostic factors for recurrence, progression, and disease-specific mortality in T1G3 bladder cancer patients treated with bacillus Calmette-Guerin. Eur Urol. 2012;62(1):118-25. Epub 2011/11/22.

[62] Lebret T, Neuzillet Y. Indication and timing of cystectomy in high-risk bladder cancer. Curr Opin Urol. 2012;22(5):427-31. Epub 2012/07/21.

[63] AUA. Bladder Cancer Clinical Guideline Update Panel (2007). Bladder Cancer: Guideline for the Management of Nonmuscle Invasive Bladder Cancer: (Stages

Ta,T1, and Tis): 2007 Update. American Urology Association; 2007 [cited 2012 August 15th]; Available from: http://www.auanet.org/content/clinical-practice-guidelines/clinical-guidelines.cfm?sub=bc.

[64] Babjuk M, Oosterlinck W, Sylvester R, Kaasinen E, Bohle A, Palou-Redorta J, et al. EAU guidelines on non-muscle-invasive urothelial carcinoma of the bladder, the 2011 update. Eur Urol. 2011;59(6):997-1008. Epub 2011/04/05.

Chapter 5

Autologous Immunotherapy as a Novel Treatment for Bladder Cancer

Martin C. Schumacher and Amir M. Sherif

Additional information is available at the end of the chapter

http://dx.doi.org/10.5772/54226

1. Introduction

Cancer is fundamentally a disease with failure in regulation in tissue growth and the risk of developing cancer increases with age. The armamentarium in treating cancer is mainly threefold: surgical resection of the tumor, radiation therapy and cytotoxic drugs. For bladder cancer, results from contemporary radical cystectomy series with pelvic lymph node dissection for T2-4 NX M0 transitional cell carcinoma (TCC) provides accurate pathologic staging of the primary tumor and lymph nodes, and due to increasing expertise with the different types of urinary diversions durable preservation of quality of life. However, the 5-year survival rate for all patients with pT2 tumors is approximately 50 – 80%, and for those with negative lymph nodes 64 – 86% (Stein, Lieskovsky et al. 2001) (Shariat, Karakiewicz et al. 2006) (Hautmann, de Petriconi et al.). In contrast, the 5-year survival rates for locally advanced cancers, pT3 and pT4, in contemporary cystectomy series range from 22 – 58%. The presence of pathologically proven lymph node metastases at radical cystectomy is associated with a poor outcome with a 5-year survival of 30%.

After more than 30 years of clinically research in bladder cancer, the true role of neoadjuvant and adjuvant chemotherapy for locally advanced bladder cancer remains unclear. Neoadjuvant chemotherapy has been shown to help for debulking and facilitation for surgical resection at radical cystectomy. The overall survival benefit is unfortunately relatively low (< 9%) and treatment protocols are often not suitable in older patients with comorbidities and decreased renal function (Grossman, Natale et al. 2003) (Sonpavde, Amiel et al. 2008) (2005). Identification of responders versus non-responders to neoadjuvant chemotherapy seems to be of value for selection of patients to be treated with this modality, still at present - robust and readily available markers predicting treatment response are lacking (Rosenblatt, Sherif et al.). Adjuvant chemotherapy trials have been less clear, with at least a trend of improved disease-free survival in small series of statistically underpowered trials (Walz, Shariat et al. 2008). Thus, other treatment modalities are highly warranted for these patients.

Immunotherapy offers an appealing complement to traditional chemotherapy, with possible long-term protection against tumor recurrences through immunological memory. Vaccination trials have shown promising results in colorectal cancer patients (Hanna, Hoover et al. 2001) (Mocellin, Rossi et al. 2004) (Karlsson, Marits et al.). Similar studies have been performed in patients with malignant melanoma (Dudley, Wunderlich et al. 2005). Adoptive immunotherapy with the collection and expansion of autologous tumor-reactive lymphocytes, followed by re-transfusion to the patient, has been reported to influence tumor progression. Another approach, using a combination between adoptive immunotherapy and a retroviral gene therapy using specific malignant melanoma T cell receptors, showed sustained levels of circulating, engineered cells at one year after infusion in two patients who both demonstrated objective regression of metastatic melanoma lesions (Morgan, Dudley et al. 2006).

Due to promising results using adoptive immunotherapy, our interests turned to bladder cancer, as few new cytotoxic drugs are available. This review provides an overview on the concept of sentinel node detection, necessary for the collection and expansion of autologous tumor-reactive lymphocytes in bladder cancer patients, as a novel adoptive immunotherapy.

2. Immunotherapy as cancer therapy

Over the past decade, interest has turned to other treatment concepts as novel cancer strategies than cytotoxic drugs. A variety of immunotherapeutic approaches have been tested in order to stimulate the cellular and humoral arms of the immune system to induce tumor regression. Currently, the following treatment strategies seem most promising, including the application of cytokines and adjuvant agents which modulate the cytokine response, cancer vaccines designed to elicit cellular immune responses against tumor associated antigens (TAAs), and monoclonal antibody drugs (Kusmartsev and Vieweg 2009).

Despite better understanding of the immune system only a few immunotherapeutic approaches have received approval by the Federal Drug Agency (FDA) for treatment of urological malignancies, such as the systemic administration of interleukin (IL-2) against metastatic renal cell cancer (RCC) and the intravesical instillation of bacillus Calmette-Guérin (BCG) or interferon α for non-muscle-invasive bladder cancer. The cancer vaccine that has received the most publicity and attention is undoubtedly Sipuleucel-T or Provenge® (Lubaroff 2012). The vaccine was approved by the FDA in April 2010 for men with asymptomatic or minimal symptomatic castration resistant prostate cancer (CRPC).

Cancer vaccines are designed to stimulate expansion of the cellular arm of the immune system, mainly T cells and natural killer cells. Cytotoxic and helper T lymphocytes are considered the main immune effector cells, which in turn kill tumor cells via receptor mediated interactions. Both cell types require activation by antigen presenting cells, such as dendritic cells (DCs), to recognize and kill tumor cells in context with major histocompatibility complex (MHC) self-antigens. Natural killer cells, by contrast, kill rather non-specifically and represent the first line of immunological defense against cancer and foreign pathogens. Many vaccine approaches have shown high efficacy at triggering T-cell responses against TAAs in tumor bearing animals—these approaches include vaccination with gene modified tumor cells, antigen-loaded DCs, recombinant viral expression cassettes, and heat shock proteins (Kusmartsev and Vieweg 2009).

Despite the fact that many immunologic approaches have moved from basic research into clinical trials, only a few showed clinical response and tumor regression. As the rates of tumor regression has seldom exceeded 5 - 10%, with only a short duration of clinical response, the efficacy of these treatments has been seriously questioned (Vieweg and Dannull 2005). A possible explanation for the limited response of cancer vaccines lies in the fact that new drugs must be initially studied in patients with advanced or metastatic disease, with poor survival outcome. Additionally, the immunogenicity of the TAAs used in reported vaccine formulations is low, as most TAAs represent self-antigens that are overexpressed or reactivated in cancer cells relative to the non-cancerous cells from which they originated. Finally, tumors can evade the immune system (including the immune responses triggered by vaccination) through the induction of immune tolerance or immune suppression (Kusmartsev and Vieweg 2009) (Gilboa 2004) (Rabinovich, Gabrilovich et al. 2007).

In times of economic uncertainties, cancer vaccine treatments are not without controversy. The controversial issues that have been raised in using Sipuleucel-T include the high cost, the modest improvement in overall survival (OS) and virtually an absence of change in time to progression (Chambers and Neumann 2011) (Goozner 2011). Priced at $31,000 per treatment, with a usual course of three treatments, Sipuleucel-T is one of the most expensive cancer therapies ever to hit the marketplace. Whether, health care providers can afford these additional burden remains to be seen in the near future.

3. Immunotherapy in non-advanced urothelial carcinoma

Bladder cancer is the fifth most commonly diagnosed cancer in the US in 2012 (after prostate, breast, lung, and colon cancers), with an estimated 73'510 new cases and 14'880 deaths (2012). Risk factors for developing bladder cancer include cigarette smoking, exposure to arsenic, occupation in rubber or fossil oil industry, and schistosomiasis, and chronic inflammatory disease (Steineck, Plato et al. 1990). Approximately 70% to 80% of patients with newly diagnosed bladder cancer will present as noninvasive papillary transitional-cell carcinomas (TCCs), 70% of which will recur, and 10 – 20% of which will progress and invade the bladder wall (Babjuk, Oosterlinck et al. 2012). Those who do present with superficial, noninvasive bladder cancer can often be cured, and those with deeply invasive disease can sometimes be cured by surgery, radiation therapy, or a combination of modalities that include chemotherapy.

According to the National Cancer Institute's Surveillance Epidemiology and End Results (SEER) registry, there has been a gradually increasing incidence of bladder cancer over the past three decades (Kamel, Moore et al.). The incidence of muscle invasive tumors has remained stable over this time; however, the incidence of superficial, noninvasive bladder cancer is rising.

Transurethral resection of bladder tumor (TURBT) is the standard initial therapeutic approach for diagnosis and treatment of nonmuscle invasive bladder cancer (NMIBC) (Babjuk, Oosterlinck et al. 2012) (Williams, Hoenig et al. 2010) (Brausi, Witjes et al.). However, although TURBT is an effective therapy, up to 45% of patients will experience tumor recurrence within 1 year after TURBT alone (Hall, Chang et al. 2007). Additionally, a 3 to 15% risk of tumor progression to muscle-invasive and/or metastatic cancer has been reported. According to these figures TURBT alone is considered to be an insufficient treatment modality in most patients. To overcome the limitations of TURBT alone, interest has turned towards adjuvant intravesical treatment regimens since the early 1970s.

The difficulty in the management of bladder cancer comes from the inability to predict which tumors will recur or progress. Current evidence suggest for the existence of mutually exclusive molecular pathways to tumorigenesis, responsible for the formation of papillary and invasive carcinomas, respectively (Wolff, Liang et al. 2005). The most common genetic alterations in low grade papillary TCC are loss of heterozygosity of part or all of chromosome 9 and activating mutations of the fibroblast growth factor receptor 3 (*FGFR3*) (Cappellen, De Oliveira et al. 1999; Cheng, Huang et al. 2002; Bakkar, Wallerand et al. 2003). In contrast to the pathway responsible for the development of invasive TCC which seems to start with dysplasia, progress to carcinoma *in situ*, followed by invasion of the lamina propria. The most frequent genetic alteration in dysplasia and carcinoma *in situ* is mutation of *TP53*, followed by loss of heterozygosity of chromosome 9 (Burkhard, Markwalder et al. 1997; Orlow, LaRue et al. 1999; Sarkar, Julicher et al. 2000; Hartmann, Schlake et al. 2002). An important marker for progression in TCC is loss of chromosome 8p, which occurs in approximately 60% of bladder tumors (Stoehr, Wissmann et al. 2004). Global trends of increased genomic instability and aberrant methylation of cytosine residues in DNA correlate with increased tumor invasion and progression (Dulaimi, Uzzo et al. 2004). This may partly explain why the incidence of superficial, noninvasive bladder cancer is rising (Kamel, Moore et al.).

4. Intravesical immunotherapy

Bacillus Calmette-Guerin (BCG) is the most commonly used first-line immunotherapeutic agent for prophylaxis and treatment of carcinoma in situ and high-grade bladder cancer. BCG has fundamentally changed the management of high risk nonmuscle invasive TCC, particularly carcinoma in situ (CIS) (Babjuk, Oosterlinck et al.). The aim of adjuvant intravesical immunotherapy is to avoid post-TURBT implantation of tumor cells, eradicate residual cancer cells and delay tumor recurrence by local immunostimulation (Soloway, Nissenkorn et al. 1983). The effect on cancer progression is unclear.

Other immunotherapeutic drugs include the interferons (IFN), interleukin (IL-2, IL-12), as well as tumor necrosis factor (TNF), which have their place in BCG-refractory patients (Glazier, Bahnson et al. 1995; Magno, Melloni et al. 2002; Weiss, O'Donnell et al. 2003).

5. Bacillus Calmette-Guerin (BCG)

BCG is a live-attenuated vaccine, and until today considered to be the most effective intravesical treatment for carcinoma in situ and high grade stage Ta or T1 TCC (Shelley, Kynaston et al. 2001; Han and Pan 2006). It was developed by Albert Calmette and Camille Guerin in 1921 at the Pasteur Institute in France by attenuating the bovine tuberculous bacillus, Mycobacterium bovis (Calmette 1931; Herr and Morales 2008). The background of the antitumor properties of BCG is based on observational autopsy studies in tuberculosis patients which had a lower frequency of various tumors (Pearl 1929). Old et al. were the first to demonstrate a potential benefit using BCG in infected mice who showed increased resistance to challenge with transplantable tumors (Old, Clarke et al. 1959). Ten years later Mathe et al. reported encouraging results with BCG as adjuvant therapy for acute lymphoblastic leukemia (Mathe, Pouillart et al. 1969). In 1976, Morales et al. were the first to report the successful use of BCG in the treatment of bladder cancer (Morales, Eidinger et al. 1976).

The exact mechanisms of action and its antitumor properties of BCG in bladder cancer remains to be elucidated. However, immediately after intravesical instillation, BCG infects and is internalized into urothelial and bladder cancer cells via a fibronectin-dependent process mediated by integrins (Becich, Carroll et al. 1991; Kuroda, Brown et al. 1993). Fibronectin attachment protein (FAP) mediates BCG attachment to bladder cancer cells and the urothelial wall following intravesical instillation. The interaction between BCG with urothelial cells results in several immunologically changes, including induction of chemokines such as interleukin (IL)-1, IL-6, IL-8, IL-17 [18], GM-CSF, tumor necrosis factor (TNF), and the up-regulation of intracellular adhesion molecule (ICAM)-1 (Alexandroff, Jackson et al. 1999; Simons, O'Donnell et al. 2008). These cytokines are considered critical for cellular assault by causing tumor cells to display molecules that serve as attachment anchors for immune cells, including neutrophils and T lymphocytes, and activation signals such as ICAM-1, fatty-acid synthetase (FAS), CD40, *etc* (Alexandroff, Jackson et al. 1999; Wolff, Liang et al. 2005). The importance of these immunologic changes can be partly assessed by the high level of IL-8 production which is associated with better clinical responses to BCG (Thalmann, Dewald et al. 1997; Thalmann, Sermier et al. 2000).

After weekly intravesical instillations of BCG, a variety of immune cells such as neutrophils, macrophages, natural killer cells, T lymphocytes, and NKT cells are constantly recruited. Urinary samples from patients under BCG instillation therapy contain almost seventy-five percent of neutrophils, five to ten percent of macrophages and one to three percent of NK cells (De Boer, De Jong et al. 1991). The neutrophils secrete cytokines which in turn activate various effector cells. To achieve an immunologic reaction and a potential therapeutic effect it takes five to six BCG instillations (Prescott, James et al. 1992) (Jackson, Alexandroff et al. 1995).

Potential effector cells responsible for tumor killing include MHC-nonrestricted cells such as NK cells lymphokine-activated killer (LAK) cells, BCG-activated killer cells, CD-1-restricted CD8+ T cells, gd T cells, NKT cells, neutrophils, macrophages, and MHC-restricted CD8+ and CD4+ T cells (Kitamura and Tsukamoto 2011). Of these cells, T lymphocytes are considered to be the most effective effector cells responsible for eliminating cancer cells (Alexandroff, Nicholson et al.). In a depletion study, both CD8+ and CD4+ T cells were found to be essential for the successful antitumor effects of BCG (Ratliff, Ritchey et al. 1993).

According to the current literature at least four meta-analyses have shown that TURBT plus intravesical BCG is superior to TURBT alone for delaying time to first tumor recurrence (Shelley, Kynaston et al. 2001; Bohle and Bock 2004; Shelley, Wilt et al. 2004; Han and Pan 2006). The largest meta-analysis by the EORTC reviewed data from 24 randomized trials and reported that the progression rate in the group TURBT plus BCG was 9.8% vs. 13.8% in the control groups with a median follow-up of 2.5 years (maximum up to 15 years) (Pawinski, Sylvester et al. 1996). Despite the fact that BCG may delay tumor progression, patients are still at risk for metastatic or muscle-invasive disease. This has been highlighted in the study by Lamm et al. on the natural history of untreated CIS with a progression rate to muscle-invasive disease in 54% (Lamm 1992).

Even with initial complete response after BCG treatment regimens, there is a continued risk for tumor recurrence or the occurrence of new tumors on the long-term. Thus, according to the risk assessment of the tumor lifelong surveillance is mandatory.

The administration of intravesical BCG, as well as its optimum dose and treatment schedule remains under investigation. Until today the original treatment protocol by Morales et al. of six instillations, once a week for six weeks, is still considered standard of care (Morales, Eidinger et al. 1976). Cystoscopy with urinary cytology is performed six weeks after completion of BCG instillation to assess treatment response (Babjuk, Oosterlinck et al.).

6. Interferons (INFs)

IFNs are host-produced glycoproteins which act to mediate immune responses through antiviral, antiproliferative, and immuneregulatory activities (Williams, Hoenig et al.). In vitro studies have shown that INFs have direct antitumor effects (Baron, Tyring et al. 1991). INF-α2b has been the most extensively studied interferon as an intravesical agent, and it seems that the in vitro effect of antiproliferative activity on bladder cancer cells are also observed in vivo (Molto, Alvarez-Mon et al. 1995). Several studies comparing the antitumor activity of INF-α2b com-

http://dx.doi.org/10.5772/54226

pared with BCG, demonstrated a clear inferiority regarding risk for recurrence or time to first recurrence (Kalble, Beer et al. 1994; Portillo, Martin et al. 1997). For this reason, and the high costs of INF-α2b, INF-α2b has been mainly used for salvage treatment protocols, as BCG failure patients have a 15 - 20% complete response to INF-α2b at one year (Lam, Benson et al. 2003).

In order to determine whether mitomycin C followed by BCG vs. BCG plus IFN-a2b decreased the intravesical recurrence rate, a randomized study could demonstrate that there is no benefit by alternating IFN-a2b with BCG (Kaasinen, Rintala et al. 2000). Thus addition of IFN-a to BCG does not seem to enhance the antitumor effects of BCG immunotherapy.

7. Future perspectives for intravesical treatments

Besides urgent need for tumor markers in bladder cancer patients to better detect recurrences, attempts are under investigation for optimal drug delivery using intravesical treatments. Different devices are currently under investigation such as thermochemotherapy and electromotive drug administration in non-muscle invasive bladder tumors. The idea behind these drug delivery approaches is to temporarily breach the urothelium which in turn should lead in an increased accumulation of drugs in the bladder tissue. First results are encouraging using electromotive mitomycin C (eMMC) instillations in patients with CIS, with a statistically significant, superior complete response rate at 6 months for eMMC (58%) compared to passive MMC at the higher doses (31%) (Di Stasi, Giannantoni et al. 2003). The response rate of eMMC approached that of BCG (64%). Local microwave hyperthermia (Synergo system) is another technology being investigated in the treatment of bladder cancer. The Synergo system stimulates bladder wall hyperthermia through an energy delivering unit in the tip of a special catheter equipped with internal thermocouples designed to maintain temperatures between 42 and 43°C. The aim is to increases cell-membrane permeability and by this way alter intracellular drug trafficking and distribution (Moskovitz, Meyer et al. 2005). Whether these combined approaches using thermal energy and intravesical agents will revolutionize the treatment of bladder cancer remains to be seen in the future (Williams, Hoenig et al. 2010).

Another approach has been reported by Sharma et al. in a post TURBT adjuvant setting (Sharma, Bajorin et al. 2008). The safety and immunogenicity of a recombinant NY-ESO-1 protein vaccine, which was administered with granulocyte macrophage colony-stimulating factor and BCG as immunologic adjuvant was tested in a cohort of urothelial carcinoma patients. Six patients met all eligibility criteria to receive the vaccination after TURBT for localized TCC. Tumor tissues were tested for NY-ESO-1 expression and patients, shown to have NY-ESO-1 tumors, were vaccinated in the postoperative setting. Peripheral blood samples were analyzed for vaccine-induced antibody and T-cell responses. NY-ESO-1-specific antibody responses were induced in 5/6 patients whereas CD8 T-cell responses occurred in 1/6 patients and CD4 T-cell responses were found in 6/6 patients. This study demonstrates safety and feasibility of the NY-ESO-1 recombinant protein in combination with BCG and granulocyte macrophage colony-stimulating factor to induce predominantly antibody and CD4 T-cell responses in urothelial carcinoma patients. Induction of higher frequency of CD8 T-cell responses may be possible in clinical trials implementing NY-ESO-1 vaccination in combination with other immunomodulatory agents (Sharma, Bajorin et al. 2008).

8. Sentinel lymph node concept, detection and clinical implications

The sentinel node (SN) is defined as the first tumor-draining lymph node along the direct drainage route from the tumor; in case of dissemination, it is considered being the first site of metastasis. A tumor can have more than one primary sentinel node, due to different sections of the tumor being drained. In a defined micro-anatomical drainage route, the first node is called the first echelon SN followed by the second echelon SN, the third and so forth (figure 1). Identification and subsequent pathologic examination of the SNs reflects the nodal status of the remaining regional nodes. It is postulated that regional nodes in the vicinity, which are unconnected to the tumor draining routes, by definition cannot be or become hosts of tumor dissemination. The concept of a sentinel node was first described 1960, in a patient with cancer of the parotid gland (Gould, Winship et al. 1960). Detection of the SN was further introduced in urology by Cabanas in 1977, aiming at improved accuracy in penile carcinoma staging (Cabanas 1977). The SN technique is now established as a routine method in malignant melanoma and breast cancer. SN detection is still experimental in urologic malignancies and is previously described in urinary bladder cancer (Sherif, De La Torre et al. 2001) (Sherif, Garske et al. 2006) (Liedberg, Chebil et al. 2006), in prostate cancer (Wawroschek, Vogt et al. 1999) (Jeschke, Nambirajan et al. 2005), in testicular cancer (Ohyama, Chiba et al. 2002) and in renal cell carcinoma (Sherif, Eriksson et al.) (Bex, Vermeeren et al.). A further extension of the concept is in identification of Metinel nodes (MN), which are defined as lymph nodes draining a metastatic site (Dahl, Karlsson et al. 2008). This might have further implications in subsequent immunological therapies based on using tumor extract as antigen source, due to the presence of intratumor heterogeneity both in primary tumors (Gerlinger, Rowan et al.) and the suggested clonal differentiation displayed in metastatic sites (Malmstrom, Ren et al. 2002).

Various procedures entailing/techniques for sentinel node detection:

- Preoperative planar lymphoscintigraphy
- Preoperative planar lymphoscintigraphy in conjunction with SPECT/CT [single photonemission CT (SPECT) with a low-dose CT]
- Intraoperative visual blue dye detection
- Intraoperative gamma probe/Geiger meter-detection
- Postoperative scintigraphy of main specimen with planar acquisition

In most centers one, two or three methods combined are considered being sufficient for the everyday clinical praxis.

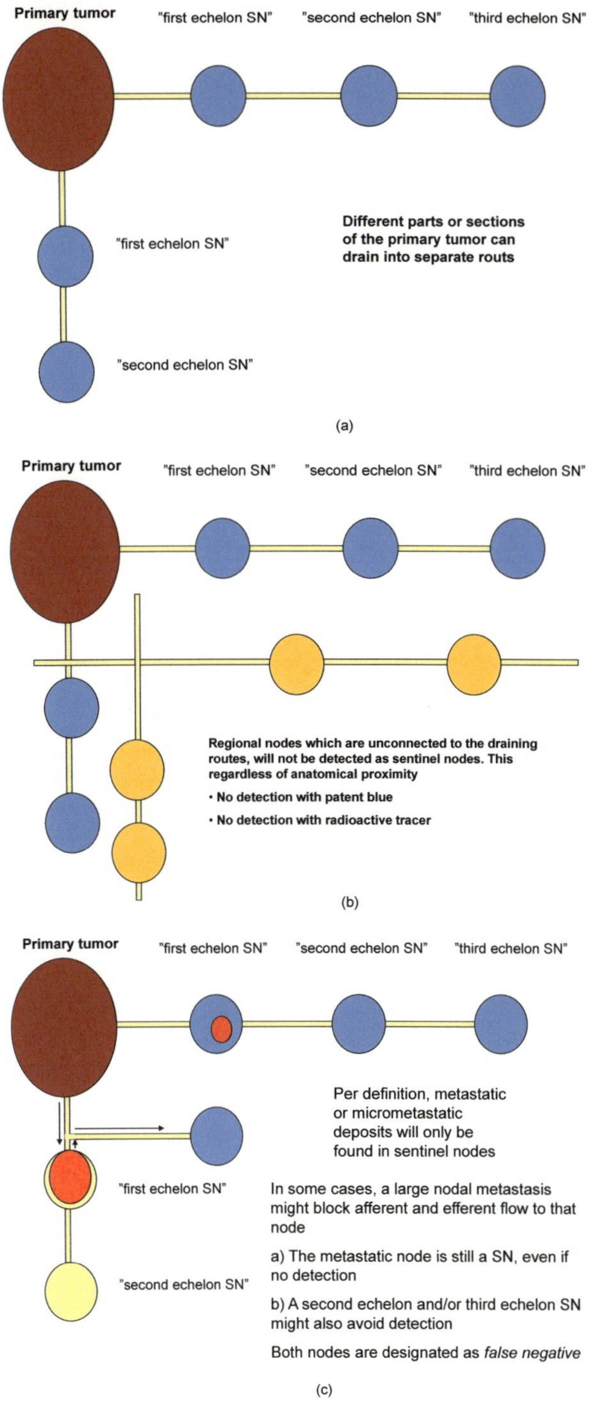
Primary tumor
"first echelon SN"
"second echelon SN"
"third echelon SN"
"first echelon SN"
Different parts or sections of the primary tumor can drain into separate routs
"second echelon SN"
(a)
Primary tumor
"first echelon SN"
"second echelon SN"
"third echelon SN"
Regional nodes which are unconnected to the draining routes, will not be detected as sentinel nodes. This regardless of anatomical proximity
• No detection with patent blue
• No detection with radioactive tracer
(b)
Primary tumor
"first echelon SN"
"second echelon SN"
"third echelon SN"
Per definition, metastatic or micrometastatic deposits will only be found in sentinel nodes
"first echelon SN"
In some cases, a large nodal metastasis might block afferent and efferent flow to that node
a) The metastatic node is still a SN, even if no detection
"second echelon SN"
b) A second echelon and/or third echelon SN might also avoid detection
Both nodes are designated as false negative
(c)

Figure 1.

9. T-cell function, including receptor and antigen recognition

The subset of lymphocytes called T cells mature in the thymus and are distinguished from other lymphocytes (B-cells, NK-cells) by their T cell receptor (TCR) located on the cell surface. Different subsets of T cells display a variety of different functions:

- T helper cell (T_H cells) [also known as CD4 cells]
- Cytotoxic T cells (CTLs or T_C) [also known as CD8 cells]
- Memory T cells
  - Central memory T cells (T_{CM} cells)
  - Effector memory T cells (T_{EM} cells)
- Regulatory T cells (T_{reg} cells)
  - Naturally occurring T_{reg} cells
  - Adaptive T_{reg} cells
- Natural killer T cells (NKT cells)
- $\gamma\delta$ T cells (gamma delta T cells)

The origin of all T cells is the hematopoietic stem cells in the bone marrow. Immature thymocytes do not express any of the two markers CD4 or CD 8. During the development of the thymocytes, they finally become either of the two major subsets followed by release to peripheral tissues. Prior to the release, the TCR has developed on the surface through different selection processes in the thymus, enabling the future mature T cell to interact with MHC/HLA complexes and also to have attained a balanced reaction to self-antigens. The T cells which exit the thymus are designated as *mature naive T cells*. The TCR is composed of two separate peptide chains joined in a complex with CD3-proteins. When the TCR is activated a number of processes take place finalizing in activation of the transcription factor NFAT (Nuclear factor of activated T-cells). NFAT translocates to the nucleus of the T cell and activates a number of genes as for instance IL-2, leading to growth, proliferation, and differentiation of the T cell. The TCR requests co-stimulation of CD28 also expressed on the T cell, for activation. In absence of interaction with CD28 when the T cell encounters APCs (antigen presenting cells), the T cell will not proliferate and the end result will be anergy and a suboptimal immunoresponse.

10. T-cell activation in lymph nodes

Animal models indicate that tumor antigensensitization of lymphocytes takes place in tumor draining lymph nodes (SNs and MNs), where tumor antigens are presented to T cells by specialized APCs (Itano and Jenkins 2003). Naive T lymphocytes are activated through their TCRs by peptide–MHC complexes displayed on dendritic cells in secondary lymphoid tissue (Jenkins, Khoruts et al. 2001). Upon activation, T cells undergo rapid proliferation, differentiating into effectors capable of migrating into various sites and of producing lymphokines. A contraction phase then results in the elimination of the vast majority of T cells, leaving behind a stable population of memory cells (Seder and Ahmed 2003).

11. Sentinel lymph node concept and immunology

In the sentinel nodes or metinel nodes, the antigen-presenting cells (most often dendritic cells) encounter tumor antigen, which is digested to peptides. The peptides are directed to the class 2 pocket and displayed on the cell surface for recognition by CD4+ T cells. Newly arrived T cells are guided to the T-cell zones of the node mainly by the chemokine CCL 21 through binding of the receptor CCR7 on the lymphocytes (Campbell, Bowman et al. 1998). On encountering the APCs, the naive T cells are specifically activated and undergo a clonal expansion.

Whereas effector memory cells are capable of executing immediate effector functions upon antigen encounter, central memory cells home to lymph nodes, may provide a lifelong source of new effector cells, both upon secondary stimulation and under the influence of homeostatic cytokines (Geginat, Sallusto et al. 2001) (Hammarlund, Lewis et al. 2003).

The tumor has its own line of defence when encountering an immunological assault in which is known as *tumor escape mechanisms*; thus tumor cells may escape elimination by losing targeted antigens, rendering T-cells anergic by downregulation of costimulatory molecules, by inducing regulatory T-lymphocytes (T-regs), or by specifically deleting responding T-lymphocytes (Staveley-O'Carroll, Sotomayor et al. 1998) (Woo, Yeh et al. 2002) (Engelhard, Bullock et al. 2002) (Lee, Yee et al. 1999).

12. Adoptive immunotherapy using autologous T-cells in bladder cancer: Results from the Karolinska University Hospital

Until now, only two pilot projects in humans describing immunotherapy using autologous T-cells collected from tumor draining lymph nodes followed by cell culture and expansion, have been published. The first one in advanced colon cancer and the second one in advanced urothelial bladder cancer. In 2006 our group described the possibility and the techniques of identifying, harvesting, enhancing, refining and multiplying mainly T helper cells (CD4+ Th1-lymphocytes) from draining sentinel lymph nodes in both colon cancer (Marits, Karlsson et al. 2006) and in bladder cancer (Marits, Karlsson et al. 2006). From there, the next step was taken and a treatment series of 16 patients with advanced colon cancer included between 2003-2008, were described (Karlsson, Nilsson et al. 2008). The selected patients were histopathologically classified as stage II, III or IV (AJCC criteria) tumors. The patients were followed for 36 months on average (range 6–51 months) and monitored in accordance with the Swedish colorectal cancer follow-up protocol. The patients with distant metastases (stage IV) responded to treatment, either with extended periods of stable disease (n = 4), partial response with diminished tumor burden (n = 1) or complete response with no detectable remaining tumor (n = 4). The cumulative survival of the nine treated stage IV patients was compared with all stage IV cases in the Stockholm region during the year of 2003. The median survival of stage IV patients receiving immunotherapy was 2.6 years compared with 0.8 years median survival of the control group.

The same approach was used in urinary bladder cancer patients and the techniques and methods were published 2010 in the first 12 patients in an ongoing pilot trial (Sherif, Hasan et al. 2010). The preliminary results have so far included a total of 18 patients, in which 9 patients received intended treatment. Two of the nine treated patients showed objective responses by RECIST criteria, and also exceptionally long overall survival (Sherif et al 2011). Further evaluation and long-term follow-up results are necessary to assess the role of immunotherapy in bladder cancer patients.

13. Future perspectives

Recent research has suggested that chemotherapy in the traditional form not only exerts its effect on different moments in the cell cycle further leading to apoptosis, but also primarily and secondarily plays a major role in tumor immunological events (Demaria, Volm et al. 2001) (Hong, Puaux et al.) (Ramakrishnan, Huang et al.). A challenging option would be to combine neoadjuvant chemotherapy in high risk groups (non-responders and partial responders to cisplatine combination therapies) with adjuvant immunotherapy in one form or another. Hypothetically, neoadjuvant chemotherapy in urinary bladder cancer could be followed by sentinel node detection in conjunction with intended cystectomy. Primarily non-responders (>pT0) could be offered inclusion in a trial entailing treatment with autologous tumor-reactive lymphocytes.

14. Summary

According to the growing body of evidence in the understanding of molecular pathways in tumor biology, other treatment modalities than surgery, chemotherapy and radiotherapy will certainly increase our possibilities to treat various cancers. Immunotherapy provides the most exciting aspect for clinical research in the near future. As these treatments are mainly applied to patients with advanced diseases it remains to be seen whether early treatment strategy immunotherapy protocols will change the course of many diseases in the near future. To date, however, there have been only a few published phase I or II clinical trials of active immunotherapy for bladder cancer (table 1) (Sharma, Bajorin et al. 2008) (Honma, Kitamura et al. 2009) (Sherif, Hasan et al. 2010) (Malmstrom, Loskog et al.) (Matsumoto, Noguchi et al.).

http://dx.doi.org/10.5772/54226

Author	Treatment protocol	Disease stage	Number of patients	Phase study	Results	Side effects
Sharma et al. [2008]	NY-ESO-1 protein vaccine + CM-CSF + BCG	Adjuvant treatment post-TURBT	6	I	Ag-specific antibodies in 5/6 pts., CD8 T cell response in 1/6 Pts, CD4 T cell response in 6/6 pts.	Only mild injection site reactions
Honma et al. [2009]	Survivin-2B80-8 8 peptide vaccination	Advanced TCC	9	I	CD8 T cell response in 5/9 pts., tumor reduction in 1/9 pts.	No side effects
Sherif et al. [2010]	Reinfusion of autologous T-helper cells	T2-T4 N1-2 M0-1 bladder cancer	12	I	Feasible in 6/12 Pts, technical failure in 6/12 Pts,	No severe adverse events
Malmström et al. [2010]	Adenoviral vector expressing CD40 ligand (intravesical)	Muscle-invasive TCC scheduled for cystectomy (phase I), Ta disease (phase II)	8	I/II	Enhancement of T cell infiltration and IFN-γ production, reduction of circulating regulatory T-cells	No severe adverse events, minor local pain
Matsumoto et al. [2011]	Personalized peptide vaccine	Advanced TCC (MVAC failure)	10	I	1 CR, 1 PR, 2 SD, PFS 3.0 months, OS 8.9 months	No severe adverse events

MVAC: methotrexate,vinblastine, adriamycin and cisplatin; CR: complete response; PR: partial response; SD: stable disease, PFS: progression-free survival; OS: overall survival

Table 1. Present phase I and II clinical trials of active immunotherapy in bladder cancer

Author details

Martin C. Schumacher[1,2] and Amir M. Sherif[1]

1 Karolinska University Hospital, Dept. of Urology, Stockholm, Sweden

2 Hirslanden Klinik Aarau, Urology, Aarau, Switzerland

References

[1] (2005). "Neoadjuvant chemotherapy in invasive bladder cancer: update of a systematic review and meta-analysis of individual patient data advanced bladder cancer (ABC) meta-analysis collaboration." Eur Urol 48(2): 202-5; discussion 205-6.

[2] (2012). "American Cancer Society.: Cancer Facts and Figures 2012. Atlanta, Ga: American Cancer Society, 2012".

[3] Alexandroff, A. B., A. M. Jackson, et al. (1999). "BCG immunotherapy of bladder cancer: 20 years on." Lancet 353(9165): 1689-94.

[4] Alexandroff, A. B., S. Nicholson, et al. (2010). "Recent advances in bacillus Calmette-Guerin immunotherapy in bladder cancer." Immunotherapy 2(4): 551-60.

[5] Babjuk, M., W. Oosterlinck, et al. (2012). "[EAU guidelines on non-muscle-invasive urothelial carcinoma of the bladder, the 2011 update]." Actas Urol Esp 36(7): 389-402.

[6] Bakkar, A. A., H. Wallerand, et al. (2003). "FGFR3 and TP53 gene mutations define two distinct pathways in urothelial cell carcinoma of the bladder." Cancer Res 63(23): 8108-12.

[7] Baron, S., S. K. Tyring, et al. (1991). "The interferons. Mechanisms of action and clinical applications." JAMA 266(10): 1375-83.

[8] Becich, M. J., S. Carroll, et al. (1991). "Internalization of bacille Calmette-Guerin by bladder tumor cells." J Urol 145(6): 1316-24.

[9] Bex, A., L. Vermeeren, et al. (2010). "Feasibility of sentinel node detection in renal cell carcinoma: a pilot study." Eur J Nucl Med Mol Imaging 37(6): 1117-23.

[10] Bohle, A. and P. R. Bock (2004). "Intravesical bacille Calmette-Guerin versus mitomycin C in superficial bladder cancer: formal meta-analysis of comparative studies on tumor progression." Urology 63(4): 682-6; discussion 686-7.

[11] Brausi, M., J. A. Witjes, et al. (2011). "A review of current guidelines and best practice recommendations for the management of nonmuscle invasive bladder cancer by the International Bladder Cancer Group." J Urol 186(6): 2158-67.

[12] Burkhard, F. C., R. Markwalder, et al. (1997). "Immunohistochemical determination of p53 overexpression. An easy and readily available method to identify progression in superficial bladder cancer?" Urol Res 25 Suppl 1: S31-5.

[13] Cabanas, R. M. (1977). "An approach for the treatment of penile carcinoma." Cancer 39(2): 456-66.

[14] Calmette, A. (1931). "Preventive Vaccination Against Tuberculosis with BCG." Proc R Soc Med 24(11): 1481-90.

[15] Campbell, J. J., E. P. Bowman, et al. (1998). "6-C-kine (SLC), a lymphocyte adhesion-triggering chemokine expressed by high endothelium, is an agonist for the MIP-3beta receptor CCR7." J Cell Biol 141(4): 1053-9.

[16] Cappellen, D., C. De Oliveira, et al. (1999). "Frequent activating mutations of FGFR3 in human bladder and cervix carcinomas." Nat Genet 23(1): 18-20.

[17] Chambers, J. D. and P. J. Neumann (2011). "Listening to Provenge--what a costly cancer treatment says about future Medicare policy." N Engl J Med 364(18): 1687-9.

[18] Cheng, J., H. Huang, et al. (2002). "Overexpression of epidermal growth factor receptor in urothelium elicits urothelial hyperplasia and promotes bladder tumor growth." Cancer Res 62(14): 4157-63.

[19] Dahl, K., M. Karlsson, et al. (2008). "Metinel node--the first lymph node draining a metastasis--contains tumor-reactive lymphocytes." Ann Surg Oncol 15(5): 1454-63.

[20] De Boer, E. C., W. H. De Jong, et al. (1991). "Presence of activated lymphocytes in the urine of patients with superficial bladder cancer after intravesical immunotherapy with bacillus Calmette-Guerin." Cancer Immunol Immunother 33(6): 411-6.

[21] Demaria, S., M. D. Volm, et al. (2001). "Development of tumor-infiltrating lymphocytes in breast cancer after neoadjuvant paclitaxel chemotherapy." Clin Cancer Res 7(10): 3025-30.

[22] Di Stasi, S. M., A. Giannantoni, et al. (2003). "Intravesical electromotive mitomycin C versus passive transport mitomycin C for high risk superficial bladder cancer: a prospective randomized study." J Urol 170(3): 777-82.

[23] Dudley, M. E., J. R. Wunderlich, et al. (2005). "Adoptive cell transfer therapy following non-myeloablative but lymphodepleting chemotherapy for the treatment of patients with refractory metastatic melanoma." J Clin Oncol 23(10): 2346-57.

[24] Dulaimi, E., R. G. Uzzo, et al. (2004). "Detection of bladder cancer in urine by a tumor suppressor gene hypermethylation panel." Clin Cancer Res 10(6): 1887-93.

[25] Engelhard, V. H., T. N. Bullock, et al. (2002). "Antigens derived from melanocyte differentiation proteins: self-tolerance, autoimmunity, and use for cancer immunotherapy." Immunol Rev 188: 136-46.

[26] Geginat, J., F. Sallusto, et al. (2001). "Cytokine-driven proliferation and differentiation of human naive, central memory, and effector memory CD4(+) T cells." J Exp Med 194(12): 1711-9.

[27] Gerlinger, M., A. J. Rowan, et al. (2012). "Intratumor heterogeneity and branched evolution revealed by multiregion sequencing." N Engl J Med 366(10): 883-92.

[28] Gilboa, E. (2004). "The promise of cancer vaccines." Nat Rev Cancer 4(5): 401-11.

[29] Glazier, D. B., R. R. Bahnson, et al. (1995). "Intravesical recombinant tumor necrosis factor in the treatment of superficial bladder cancer: an Eastern Cooperative Oncology Group study." J Urol 154(1): 66-8.

[30] Goozner, M. (2011). "Concerns about Provenge simmer as CMS ponders coverage." J Natl Cancer Inst 103(4): 288-9.

[31] Gould, E. A., T. Winship, et al. (1960). "Observations on a "sentinel node" in cancer of the parotid." Cancer 13: 77-8.

[32] Grossman, H. B., R. B. Natale, et al. (2003). "Neoadjuvant chemotherapy plus cystectomy compared with cystectomy alone for locally advanced bladder cancer." N Engl J Med 349(9): 859-66.

[33] Hall, M. C., S. S. Chang, et al. (2007). "Guideline for the management of nonmuscle invasive bladder cancer (stages Ta, T1, and Tis): 2007 update." J Urol 178(6): 2314-30.

[34] Hammarlund, E., M. W. Lewis, et al. (2003). "Duration of antiviral immunity after smallpox vaccination." Nat Med 9(9): 1131-7.

[35] Han, R. F. and J. G. Pan (2006). "Can intravesical bacillus Calmette-Guerin reduce recurrence in patients with superficial bladder cancer? A meta-analysis of randomized trials." Urology 67(6): 1216-23.

[36] Hanna, M. G., Jr., H. C. Hoover, Jr., et al. (2001). "Adjuvant active specific immunotherapy of stage II and stage III colon cancer with an autologous tumor cell vaccine: first randomized phase III trials show promise." Vaccine 19(17-19): 2576-82.

[37] Hartmann, A., G. Schlake, et al. (2002). "Occurrence of chromosome 9 and p53 alterations in multifocal dysplasia and carcinoma in situ of human urinary bladder." Cancer Res 62(3): 809-18.

[38] Hautmann, R. E., R. C. de Petriconi, et al. (2012). "Radical cystectomy for urothelial carcinoma of the bladder without neoadjuvant or adjuvant therapy: long-term results in 1100 patients." Eur Urol 61(5): 1039-47.

[39] Herr, H. W. and A. Morales (2008). "History of bacillus Calmette-Guerin and bladder cancer: an immunotherapy success story." J Urol 179(1): 53-6.

[40] Hong, M., A. L. Puaux, et al. (2011). "Chemotherapy induces intratumoral expression of chemokines in cutaneous melanoma, favoring T-cell infiltration and tumor control." Cancer Res 71(22): 6997-7009.

[41] Honma, I., H. Kitamura, et al. (2009). "Phase I clinical study of anti-apoptosis protein survivin-derived peptide vaccination for patients with advanced or recurrent urothelial cancer." Cancer Immunol Immunother 58(11): 1801-7.

[42] Itano, A. A. and M. K. Jenkins (2003). "Antigen presentation to naive CD4 T cells in the lymph node." Nat Immunol 4(8): 733-9.

[43] Jackson, A. M., A. B. Alexandroff, et al. (1995). "Changes in urinary cytokines and soluble intercellular adhesion molecule-1 (ICAM-1) in bladder cancer patients after bacillus Calmette-Guerin (BCG) immunotherapy." Clin Exp Immunol 99(3): 369-75.

[44] Jenkins, M. K., A. Khoruts, et al. (2001). "In vivo activation of antigen-specific CD4 T cells." Annu Rev Immunol 19: 23-45.

[45] Jeschke, S., T. Nambirajan, et al. (2005). "Detection of early lymph node metastases in prostate cancer by laparoscopic radioisotope guided sentinel lymph node dissection." J Urol 173(6): 1943-6.

[46] Kaasinen, E., E. Rintala, et al. (2000). "Weekly mitomycin C followed by monthly bacillus Calmette-Guerin or alternating monthly interferon-alpha2B and bacillus Calmette-Guerin for prophylaxis of recurrent papillary superficial bladder carcinoma." J Urol 164(1): 47-52.

[47] Kalble, T., M. Beer, et al. (1994). "[BCG vs interferon A for prevention of recurrence of superficial bladder cancer. A prospective randomized study]." Urologe A 33(2): 133-7.

[48] Kamel, M. H., P. C. Moore, et al. (2012). "Potential years of life lost due to urogenital cancer in the United States: trends from 1972 to 2006 based on data from the SEER database." J Urol 187(3): 868-71.

[49] Karlsson, M., P. Marits, et al. (2010). "Pilot study of sentinel-node-based adoptive immunotherapy in advanced colorectal cancer." Ann Surg Oncol 17(7): 1747-57.

[50] Karlsson, M., O. Nilsson, et al. (2008). "Detection of metastatic colon cancer cells in sentinel nodes by flow cytometry." J Immunol Methods 334(1-2): 122-33.

[51] Kitamura, H. and T. Tsukamoto (2011). "Immunotherapy for Urothelial Carcinoma: Current Status and Perspectives." cancers 3: 3055-3072.

[52] Kuroda, K., E. J. Brown, et al. (1993). "Characterization of the internalization of bacillus Calmette-Guerin by human bladder tumor cells." J Clin Invest 91(1): 69-76.

[53] Kusmartsev, S. and J. Vieweg (2009). "Enhancing the efficacy of cancer vaccines in urologic oncology: new directions." Nat Rev Urol 6(10): 540-9.

[54] Lam, J. S., M. C. Benson, et al. (2003). "Bacillus Calmete-Guerin plus interferon-alpha2B intravesical therapy maintains an extended treatment plan for superficial bladder cancer with minimal toxicity." Urol Oncol 21(5): 354-60.

[55] Lamm, D. L. (1992). "Long-term results of intravesical therapy for superficial bladder cancer." Urol Clin North Am 19(3): 573-80.

[56] Lee, P. P., C. Yee, et al. (1999). "Characterization of circulating T cells specific for tumor-associated antigens in melanoma patients." Nat Med 5(6): 677-85.

[57] Liedberg, F., G. Chebil, et al. (2006). "Intraoperative sentinel node detection improves nodal staging in invasive bladder cancer." J Urol 175(1): 84-8; discussion 88-9.

[58] Lubaroff, D. M. (2012). "Prostate cancer vaccines in clinical trials." Expert Rev Vaccines 11(7): 857-68.

[59] Magno, C., D. Melloni, et al. (2002). "The anti-tumor activity of bacillus Calmette-Guerin in bladder cancer is associated with an increase in the circulating level of interleukin-2." Immunol Lett 81(3): 235-8.

[60] Malmstrom, P. U., A. S. Loskog, et al. "AdCD40L immunogene therapy for bladder carcinoma--the first phase I/IIa trial." Clin Cancer Res 16(12): 3279-87.

[61] Malmstrom, P. U., Z. P. Ren, et al. (2002). "Early metastatic progression of bladder carcinoma: molecular profile of primary tumor and sentinel lymph node." J Urol 168(5): 2240-4.

[62] Marits, P., M. Karlsson, et al. (2006). "Sentinel node lymphocytes: tumour reactive lymphocytes identified intraoperatively for the use in immunotherapy of colon cancer." Br J Cancer 94(10): 1478-84.

[63] Marits, P., M. Karlsson, et al. (2006). "Detection of immune responses against urinary bladder cancer in sentinel lymph nodes." Eur Urol 49(1): 59-70.

[64] Mathe, G., P. Pouillart, et al. (1969). "Active immunotherapy of L1210 leukaemia applied after the graft of tumour cells." Br J Cancer 23(4): 814-24.

[65] Matsumoto, K., M. Noguchi, et al. "A phase I study of personalized peptide vaccination for advanced urothelial carcinoma patients who failed treatment with methotrexate, vinblastine, adriamycin and cisplatin." BJU Int 108(6): 831-8.

[66] Mocellin, S., C. R. Rossi, et al. (2004). "Colorectal cancer vaccines: principles, results, and perspectives." Gastroenterology 127(6): 1821-37.

[67] Molto, L., M. Alvarez-Mon, et al. (1995). "Use of intracavitary interferon-alpha-2b in the prophylactic treatment of patients with superficial bladder cancer." Cancer 75(11): 2720-6.

[68] Morales, A., D. Eidinger, et al. (1976). "Intracavitary Bacillus Calmette-Guerin in the treatment of superficial bladder tumors." J Urol 116(2): 180-3.

[69] Morgan, R. A., M. E. Dudley, et al. (2006). "Cancer regression in patients after transfer of genetically engineered lymphocytes." Science 314(5796): 126-9.

[70] Moskovitz, B., G. Meyer, et al. (2005). "Thermo-chemotherapy for intermediate or high-risk recurrent superficial bladder cancer patients." Ann Oncol 16(4): 585-9.

[71] Ohyama, C., Y. Chiba, et al. (2002). "Lymphatic mapping and gamma probe guided laparoscopic biopsy of sentinel lymph node in patients with clinical stage I testicular tumor." J Urol 168(4 Pt 1): 1390-5.

[72] Old, L. J., D. A. Clarke, et al. (1959). "Effect of Bacillus Calmette-Guerin infection on transplanted tumours in the mouse." Nature 184(Suppl 5): 291-2.

[73] Orlow, I., H. LaRue, et al. (1999). "Deletions of the INK4A gene in superficial bladder tumors. Association with recurrence." Am J Pathol 155(1): 105-13.

[74] Pawinski, A., R. Sylvester, et al. (1996). "A combined analysis of European Organization for Research and Treatment of Cancer, and Medical Research Council randomized clinical trials for the prophylactic treatment of stage TaT1 bladder cancer. European Organization for Research and Treatment of Cancer Genitourinary Tract Cancer Cooperative Group and the Medical Research Council Working Party on Superficial Bladder Cancer." J Urol 156(6): 1934-40, discussion 1940-1.

[75] Pearl, R. (1929). "A Note on the Association of Diseases." Science 70(1808): 191-2.

[76] Portillo, J., B. Martin, et al. (1997). "Results at 43 months' follow-up of a double-blind, randomized, prospective clinical trial using intravesical interferon alpha-2b in the prophylaxis of stage pT1 transitional cell carcinoma of the bladder." Urology 49(2): 187-90.

[77] Prescott, S., K. James, et al. (1992). "Intravesical Evans strain BCG therapy: quantitative immunohistochemical analysis of the immune response within the bladder wall." J Urol 147(6): 1636-42.

[78] Rabinovich, G. A., D. Gabrilovich, et al. (2007). "Immunosuppressive strategies that are mediated by tumor cells." Annu Rev Immunol 25: 267-96.

[79] Ramakrishnan, R., C. Huang, et al. (2012). "Autophagy induced by conventional chemotherapy mediates tumor cell sensitivity to immunotherapy." Cancer Res.

[80] Ratliff, T. L., J. K. Ritchey, et al. (1993). "T-cell subsets required for intravesical BCG immunotherapy for bladder cancer." J Urol 150(3): 1018-23.

[81] Rosenblatt, R., A. Sherif, et al. (2012). "Pathologic downstaging is a surrogate marker for efficacy and increased survival following neoadjuvant chemotherapy and radical cystectomy for muscle-invasive urothelial bladder cancer." Eur Urol 61(6): 1229-38.

[82] Sarkar, S., K. P. Julicher, et al. (2000). "Different combinations of genetic/epigenetic alterations inactivate the p53 and pRb pathways in invasive human bladder cancers." Cancer Res 60(14): 3862-71.

[83] Seder, R. A. and R. Ahmed (2003). "Similarities and differences in CD4+ and CD8+ effector and memory T cell generation." Nat Immunol 4(9): 835-42.

[84] Shariat, S. F., P. I. Karakiewicz, et al. (2006). "Outcomes of radical cystectomy for transitional cell carcinoma of the bladder: a contemporary series from the Bladder Cancer Research Consortium." J Urol 176(6 Pt 1): 2414-22; discussion 2422.

[85] Sharma, P., D. F. Bajorin, et al. (2008). "Immune responses detected in urothelial carcinoma patients after vaccination with NY-ESO-1 protein plus BCG and GM-CSF." J Immunother 31(9): 849-57.

[86] Shelley, M. D., H. Kynaston, et al. (2001). "A systematic review of intravesical bacillus Calmette-Guerin plus transurethral resection vs transurethral resection alone in Ta and T1 bladder cancer." BJU Int 88(3): 209-16.

[87] Shelley, M. D., T. J. Wilt, et al. (2004). "Intravesical bacillus Calmette-Guerin is superior to mitomycin C in reducing tumour recurrence in high-risk superficial bladder cancer: a meta-analysis of randomized trials." BJU Int 93(4): 485-90.

[88] Sherif, A., M. De La Torre, et al. (2001). "Lymphatic mapping and detection of sentinel nodes in patients with bladder cancer." J Urol 166(3): 812-5.

[89] Sherif, A., U. Garske, et al. (2006). "Hybrid SPECT-CT: an additional technique for sentinel node detection of patients with invasive bladder cancer." Eur Urol 50(1): 83-91.

[90] Sherif, A., M. N. Hasan, et al. (2010). "Feasibility of T-cell-based adoptive immunotherapy in the first 12 patients with advanced urothelial urinary bladder cancer. Preliminary data on a new immunologic treatment based on the sentinel node concept." Eur Urol 58(1): 105-11.

[91] Sherif, A. M., E. Eriksson, et al. (2011). "Sentinel node detection in renal cell carcinoma. A feasibility study for detection of tumour-draining lymph nodes." BJU Int 109(8): 1134-9.

[92] Simons, M. P., M. A. O'Donnell, et al. (2008). "Role of neutrophils in BCG immunotherapy for bladder cancer." Urol Oncol 26(4): 341-5.

[93] Soloway, M. S., I. Nissenkorn, et al. (1983). "Urothelial susceptibility to tumor cell implantation: comparison of cauterization with N-methyl-N-nitrosourea." Urology 21(2): 159-61.

[94] Sonpavde, G., G. E. Amiel, et al. (2008). "Neoadjuvant chemotherapy preceding cystectomy for bladder cancer." Expert Opin Pharmacother 9(11): 1885-93.

[95] Staveley-O'Carroll, K., E. Sotomayor, et al. (1998). "Induction of antigen-specific T cell anergy: An early event in the course of tumor progression." Proc Natl Acad Sci U S A 95(3): 1178-83.

[96] Stein, J. P., G. Lieskovsky, et al. (2001). "Radical cystectomy in the treatment of invasive bladder cancer: long-term results in 1,054 patients." J Clin Oncol 19(3): 666-75.

[97] Steineck, G., N. Plato, et al. (1990). "Increased risk of urothelial cancer in Stockholm during 1985-87 after exposure to benzene and exhausts." Int J Cancer 45(6): 1012-7.

[98] Stoehr, R., C. Wissmann, et al. (2004). "Deletions of chromosome 8p and loss of sFRP1 expression are progression markers of papillary bladder cancer." Lab Invest 84(4): 465-78.

[99] Thalmann, G. N., B. Dewald, et al. (1997). "Interleukin-8 expression in the urine after bacillus Calmette-Guerin therapy: a potential prognostic factor of tumor recurrence and progression." J Urol 158(4): 1340-4.

[100] Thalmann, G. N., A. Sermier, et al. (2000). "Urinary Interleukin-8 and 18 predict the response of superficial bladder cancer to intravesical therapy with bacillus Calmette-Guerin." J Urol 164(6): 2129-33.

[101] Vieweg, J. and J. Dannull (2005). "Technology Insight: vaccine therapy for prostate cancer." Nat Clin Pract Urol 2(1): 44-51.

[102] Walz, J., S. F. Shariat, et al. (2008). "Adjuvant chemotherapy for bladder cancer does not alter cancer-specific survival after cystectomy in a matched case-control study." BJU Int 101(11): 1356-61.

[103] Wawroschek, F., H. Vogt, et al. (1999). "The sentinel lymph node concept in prostate cancer - first results of gamma probe-guided sentinel lymph node identification." Eur Urol 36(6): 595-600.

[104] Weiss, G. R., M. A. O'Donnell, et al. (2003). "Phase 1 study of the intravesical administration of recombinant human interleukin-12 in patients with recurrent superficial transitional cell carcinoma of the bladder." J Immunother 26(4): 343-8.

[105] Williams, S. K., D. M. Hoenig, et al. (2010). "Intravesical therapy for bladder cancer." Expert Opin Pharmacother 11(6): 947-58.

[106] Wolff, E. M., G. Liang, et al. (2005). "Mechanisms of Disease: genetic and epigenetic alterations that drive bladder cancer." Nat Clin Pract Urol 2(10): 502-10.

[107] Woo, E. Y., H. Yeh, et al. (2002). "Cutting edge: Regulatory T cells from lung cancer patients directly inhibit autologous T cell proliferation." J Immunol 168(9): 4272-6.

Chapter 6

Metastasis After Primary Treatment — Peri-Operative and Bladder-Preservation Therapy in Muscle Invasive Diseases

Yasuyoshi Miyata and Hideki Sakai

Additional information is available at the end of the chapter

http://dx.doi.org/10.5772/56014

1. Introduction

Bladder cancer is the seventh most prevalent cancer worldwide and the second most common genitourinary malignancy. As such, it is a significant cause of morbidity and mortality. Although 75% of patients present with non-muscle invasive bladder cancer (NMIBC) at initial diagnosis and can be managed with transurethral resection (TUR), the remaining 25% show muscle-invasive bladder cancer (MIBC) at presentation (Messing, et al., 1995). In spite of improvements in surgical technique, survival rates and outcomes for patients with MIBC are not good. Radical cystectomy is unsuccessful in approximately 50% of patients with MIBC, and the 5-year overall survival rate after radical cystectomy for MIBC is only 40%-60% (Ghoneim, et al., 1997; Stein, et al. 2001; Shariat et al., 2006 Koga et al., 2008).

For these reasons, peri-operative therapies, including neo-adjuvant and adjuvant chemotherapy, have become more prominent and have been investigated in many trials and studies (Hussain, et al., 2003; Goethuys and Van Poppel, 2012). Unfortunately, the percentages of patients receiving neo-adjuvant and adjuvant chemotherapy for locally advanced bladder cancer (T2-T4a) are only 12% and 22%, respectively (Feifer et al., 2011). One reason for the low treatment rate with these modalities is that some urologists do not prefer a conservative treatment option or to engage in a surgical approach, while others do not collaborate easily across disciplines. This paper will provide a clear, straightforward description of trends in peri-operative therapy for bladder cancer.

Organ conservation by combined modality therapy is commonplace in contemporary oncology and has achieved success in selected patients with various types of malignancies, such as breast, larynx, esophagus, and prostate. However, radical cystectomy remains the most commonly offered treatment for bladder cancer; indeed, it is sometimes performed unconditionally, even though this operation holds the possibility of significant morbidity. Modern bladder conservation approaches combine surgery, chemotherapy, and radiation therapy. However, there is variation in each protocol and in the methods used to carry out the protocols.

Over the last decade, numerous investigators have paid special attention to the multiple interacting molecular pathways in urothelial cancer cells, and have demonstrated the complex mechanisms of such interactions and their pathological roles in human bladder cancer. Previous in vivo and in vitro studies have identified several factors as key to the development and progression of urothelial cancer cells. In this paper, we highlight some of the major molecular pathways and their clinical and pathological significance in bladder cancer. We also present some molecular targeted agents and clinical trials in patients with MIBC.

2. Neo-adjuvant chemotherapy

One advantage of neo-adjuvant therapy compared with adjuvant therapy is that patient tolerance is better; this is because the therapy is administered before surgery, including before radical cystectomy. In addition, neo-adjuvant therapy allows for down-grading and down-staging, which may increase the likelihood of resectability (Calabro and Sternberg, 2009). Studies have shown that preoperative neo-adjuvant chemoradiation therapy reduced tumors to the level of pT0 in approximately one quarter to one third of patients by the time cystectomy was performed (Grossman et al., 2003; Alva et al., 2012). Such statistics give supporting evidence to the possibility that bladder conservation therapy is a practical alternative for selected patients with MIBC. This section will outline the history and present status of neo-adjuvant therapy for patients with MIBC.

There have been several key randomized trials of radical cystectomy alone or with neo-adjuvant therapy (Table 1). Among these trials, there has been no report of any single-agent regimen producing a survival benefit through neo-adjuvant therapy (Wallance et al., 1991; Martinez-Pineiro et al., 1995). A similar result was confirmed in a meta-analysis of individual data from 2688 patients enrolled in 10 randomized trials (Advanced Bladder Cancer (ABC) Meta-analysis Collaboration, 2003). On the other hand, there have been conflicting results on the survival benefit of multi-agent chemotherapy. Among them, the Nordic Cystectomy Trial I, performed using preoperative radiation therapy and 2 cycles of cisplatin (CDDP) and doxorubicin (DXR) for patients with cT1G3-T4NxM0 disease, demonstrated no survival benefit, either 5-year overall or cause-specific (Malmström et al., 1996). Similarly, the Nordic Cystectomy Trial II (3 cycles of CDDP and methotrexate, MTX) showed no overall significant difference in 5-year survival in 317 patients (Sherif et al., 2002). Thus, early trials revealed no significant survival benefit of neo-adjuvant chemotherapy. Interestingly, however, the Nordic Cystectomy Trial I also showed a 15% difference in overall survival for T3–T4a patients ($P = 0.03$). In addition, a combined analysis of the two Nordic Cystectomy Trials showed that the 5-year survival rates of patients receiving neo-adjuvant therapy (56%) were significantly better ($P = 0.049$) compared with the patients not receiving neo-adjuvant therapy (48%) (Sherif, et al.,

2004). These investigators concluded that neo-adjuvant platinum-based combination chemotherapy was associated with a 20% reduction in the relative hazard of the probability of death. In addition, a total of 449 patients form Nordic Cystectomy trial also showed that percentage of pT0N0 was nearly double in the neo-adjuvant arm compared with controls (22.7% versus 12.5%, P = 0.006). Furthermore, there is a report that CDDP, MTX, and vinblastine (VBL) showed more favorable results with neo-adjuvant chemotherapy compared with local therapy alone without neo-adjuvant therapy (Medical Research Council, 1999). On the basis of previously reported studies, one opinion is that neo-adjuvant chemotherapy cannot be regarded as standard care (Kaufman et al., 2009). On the other hand, a trial with MVAC (methotrexate, vinblastine, doxorubicin [adriamycin], and cisplatin) therapy showed a trend toward a survival benefit with MVAC, although this difference did not reach the level of significance (P = 0.06) (Grossman et al., 2003). Another prospective randomized trial by Griffiths et al. (2011) showed that neo-adjuvant chemotherapy produced a survival benefit. This study had a large impact because of the large study population (n = 976) and long follow-up periods (median and interquartile range = 8.0 and 5.7 to 10.2 years). Thus, there are contrary opinions regarding the survival benefit of neo-adjuvant chemotherapy for patients with MIBC. However, a meta-analysis of 11 randomized trials conducted by the Advanced Bladder Cancer Meta-analysis Collaboration that included 3005 bladder cancer patients demonstrated that neo-adjuvant CDDP-based therapy had a significant positive effect on the absolute 5-year overall survival rate (P = 0.003) and absolute disease-free survival rate (P < 0.0001) compared with local therapy alone. A similar finding was reported in an additional meta-analysis (Winquiest et al., 2004).

Authors (year)	Intervention	N	Clinical stage	Comments
Wallace (1991)	CDDP + Radiation therapy Radiation therapy alone	255	T2-4NxM0	No difference for overall survival (odds ratio=1.13 and 95% confidential interval=0.80-1.57)
Martinez (1995)	CDDP+Cystectomy Cystectomy alone	121	T2-4a Nx-2M0	pT0 was found in 14.3% of the experimental arm. No difference for cause-specific survival (P=0.1349).
Malmström (1996)	CDDP+ADM+Cystectomy Cystectomy alone	325	T1G3-T4aNxM0	ND for overall survival (P=0.1) in T1-2 15% benefit in T3-4a
ICT (1999)	CMV + definitive treatment Definitive treatment alone	976	T2G3-T4aN0/XM0	3-year overall survival rates were 50.0% in chemotherapy arm versus 55.5% in no-chemotherapy arm (P=0.075).
Sherif (2002)	CDDP+MTX+Cystectomy Cystectomy alone	317	T2-4a NxM0	pT0 in experimental arm was higher (26.4%) than control arm (11.5%, P=0.001). No difference for overall survival
Grossman (2003)	MVAC+Cystectomy Cystectomy alone	317	T2-4a NxM0	Pathological CR was higher in MVAC group (P<0.001). Trends in benefit for overall survival (P=0.06) .
Sherif (2004)	CDDP+ADM or CDDP+MTX +Cystectomy vs Cystectomy	620	T1G3-T4aNxM0	5-year overall survival rate were better (P=0.045) in experimental arm (56%) than that in control arm (48%).
ICT (2011)	CMV + definitive treatment Definitive treatment alone	976	T2G3-T4aN0/XM0	5-year overall survival rates were 49 versus 43% and 10-year rates were 36 versus 30% (P=0.037).

ICT: International Collaboration of Trialists

Table 1. Randomized studies for Neo-adjuvant therapy

3. Adjuvant therapy

The advantage of adjuvant chemotherapy compared with neo-adjuvant chemotherapy is that various clinical judgments can be made based on complete pathological information. This avoids over-treatment and unnecessary adverse events because pathological staging enables improved accuracy in patient selection for specific therapies. However, the anti-tumor effects and survival benefits of adjuvant chemotherapy are controversial. Several randomized prospective trials showed that adjuvant chemotherapy following cystectomy produced a survival benefit (Skinner, et al., 1991; Stockle 1995). However, these reports are relatively old (1990s) and underpowered (<100 patients). A study in 2010 by Paz et al. showed significantly longer overall survival in patients receiving adjuvant chemotherapy than in patients without adjuvant chemotherapy. Although this study had a relatively large number (n = 142), it was closed early because of slow data accrual and un-published data. Other large and recent trials (n > 100) have demonstrated that adjuvant chemotherapy following cystectomy did not show a significant survival difference compared with cystectomy alone (Stadler, et al. 2011; Cognetti, et al. 2012). Svatek (2010) conducted a large retrospective study on the relationship between adjuvant therapy and survival, and showed that adjuvant therapy (n = 932, 23.6%) was independently associated with favorable overall survival in 3947 bladder cancer patients.

As a result of such controversy, clinical trials on the survival benefit of adjuvant chemotherapy are relatively underpowered because of the small number of patients and are closed early due to poor data accrual. Another reason is the disadvantages of adjuvant chemotherapy, including post-operative complications and decrease in renal function. Donat (2009) found that approximately 30% of patients who received radical cystectomy and were candidates for adjuvant chemotherapy could not receive it within 90 days after operation. Thus, the role and aim of adjuvant chemotherapy after radical cystectomy is not clear. We close our discussion of this issue in the present paper because our main purposes are to discuss the prevention of cancer cell dissemination and understand the processes in MIBC.

4. Bladder conservation strategy

Loss of bladder function is considered a major type of mutilation. Despite advances in neobladder construction, a decrease in the quality of life (QOL) is inevitable after cystectomy. In addition, although progress has occurred in peri-operative management, radical cystectomy still has a high risk of complications, including peri-operative mortality (Manoharan, et al., 2009). A recent large review (Shansigh, et al., 2009) of 1,142 patients showed that an early complication (that is, within 90 days) occurred in 64% of patients undergoing radical cystectomy; 13% of the complications were classed as grade 3-5 by the modified Clavien grading system. In recent years, multimodality bladder conservation strategies have gradually gained popularity, and various investigations have been undertaken. In fact, an organ conservation strategy is useful to preserve bladder function and QOL (Zietman, et al., 2003). A modern bladder conservation strategy is the use of trimodality therapy, which combines maximal TUR followed by an induction course of concurrent radiotherapy and chemotherapy. Patients who incompletely respond to the combined treatment are advised to undergo immediate cystectomy. However, at present, consensus has yet to be reached on the efficacy of bladder conservation therapy for the inhibition of cancer cell progression, and prolongation of survival has yet to be reached (Herr, et al., 1998).

4.1. Present status of bladder conservation therapy

Appropriate candidates for bladder conservation therapy include: patients with T2-4a and clinically node-negative disease, proposed complete or near-complete operation, and adequate organ function to tolerate chemotherapy. Many urologists, medical oncologists, and radiation oncologists have tried various protocols to decrease local recurrence and metastasis, and to improve survival. In the beginning, various monotherapies were also investigated as a safe method of treatment. However, several key studies from pioneer centers in the 1990s to 2000s found that a combination of TUR, chemotherapy, and radiotherapy yielded more favorable outcomes and better anti-tumor effects than monotherapies and other combination therapies (Housset, 1993; Rodel, 2002; Shipley, 2002). At present, trimodality therapy is the major treatment strategy for bladder preservation. In addition, with improvements in radiation therapy and the development of chemotherapy, several trials have been performed in patients with MIBC who are clinically node-positive (Röedel et al., 2002; Gamal El-deeen et al., 2009). Furthermore, trials have also been performed in MIBC patients with multiple tumors (Zhang, et al. 2010). Thus, the applications for bladder conservation therapy are expanding. Representative reports on outcomes of bladder preservation therapies are shown in Table 2. This table lists relatively large studies (over 100 patients) on trimodality therapy, as well as randomized trials for patients with MIBC with/without lymph node metastasis. In addition to them, several interesting and important studies have been reported. For example, the protocol that radiation with combination chemotherapy of paclitaxel and CDDP chemotherapy was administrated after TUR was reported in T2-T4a bladder cancer patients. In this protocol, if repeat biopsy showed less than T1 disease, consolidation with similar chemo-radiation therapy was given. If repeat biopsy showed greater than pT1 disease, cystectomy and adjuvant GC therapy were given. Of the 80 eligible patients, 65 patients (81%) were judged complete response. However, of these 65 patients, 8 patients (28%) had local bladder recurrence. At median follow-up of 49.4 months, the actuarial 5-year overall and cause-specific survival rate was 56% and 71%, respectively. In addition, the actuarial rate of surviving with an intact bladder was 59% at 36 months and 47% at 60 months (Kaufman, et al. 2009). On the other hand, On the other hand, most recently, a large study on long-term outcomes of bladder preservation by combined-modality therapy for MIBC has also been reported from Massachusetts General Hospital (Efstathiou et al., 2012). This study showed the outcomes in 348 patients with T2-4a disease who were treated with CDDP-based chemotherapy and radiotherapy after maximal TUR plus neo-adjuvant or adjuvant therapy. Survival analysis of median follow-up at 7.7 years demonstrated that 5-, 10-, and 15-year overall survival rates were 55%, 35%, and 22%, respectively. On the other hand, the 5-, 10-, and 15-year cumulative bladder-intact disease-specific survival rates were 60%, 45%, and 36%, respectively. These investigators also showed that 102 patients (29%) required follow-up cystectomy. In the conclusion of their report, Efstathiou et al. stated their opinion that bladder conservation therapy offers a unique opportunity for urologic surgeons, radiation oncologists, and medical oncologists to work together in a truly multidisciplinary effort for the benefit of patients with invasive bladder cancer. Likewise, we and many other investigators have also suggested that the bladder conservation strategy is a useful and practical alternative for patients who are selected appropriately and when clinical management includes the methods described below.

Author (year)	N	Clinical stage	Random	Operation	Induction therapy	Consolidative therapy	Route	5 years- (%) Survival	BIS
Kachnic (1997)	106	T2-4aNxM0	No	TUR	CMV and RT+CDDP	RT+ CDDP	IV	OS: 52 CSS: 60	43
Shipley (1998)	A: 61 B: 62	T2-4aNxM0	Yes	TUR	A: CMV and RT+CDDP B: No chemotherapy	RT+ CDDP	IV	A: OS: 49 B: OS: 48	A: 38 B: 36
Rödel (2002)	415	T1-4NanyM0	No	TUR	CDDP/CBDCA±5FU+RT or RT alone	–	IV	OS: 50 CSS: 56	42
Eapen (2004)	112	Ta-4N0M0	No	TUR	CDDP+RT	–	IA	OS: 50 CSS: –	– –
Weiss (2007)	112	T1-4N0M0	No	TUR	CDDP+5FU and RT	–	IV	OS: 74 CSS: 82	61
Perdoná (2008)	43 78	T2-4N0M0	No	TUR	CMV and RT CMV and RT+CDDP	–	IV	OS: 60 OS: 72	47 54
Gamal El-Deen (2009)	114 72	T2-4aNanyM0	No	TUR	MCV/MVAC/GC and RT RT alone	–	IV	OS: 60 OS: 68	– –
Zhang (2010)	100	T2-4N0M0	No	Partial	MVAC+RT: as adjuvant for pT3+4 or pN+	–	IV	OS: – CSS: 68	– –
Sabba (2010)	104	T2-3aN0M0	No	TUR	GC and RT+CDDP	–	IV	OS: 55 CSS: –	– –

OS: Overall survival; CSS: Cause-specific survival, BIS: Bladder intact survival

Table 2. Published reports on bladder-conserving therapy (randomized study or patients number >100)

4.2. Intra-arterial chemotherapy in the bladder conservation strategy

Regarding the administration of chemotherapeutic drugs, intravenous infusion has been common in almost all of the large studies (Table 2). On the other hand, intra-arterial chemotherapy has also been used because infusion of chemotherapeutic drug(s) via the intra-arterial route enables a higher drug concentration to be directed at the primary bladder tumor. This treatment strategy, that is, the combination of intra-arterial chemotherapy and radiation therapy, has been used in several studies. For example, Eapen, et al. (1989) reported intra-arterial CDDP and concurrent radiation therapy with/without cystectomy in 25 bladder cancer patients with T3-4N0M0 disease. Another example is that our own study group reported on a combination therapy for 35 bladder cancer patients with T2-4N0M0, for whom two courses of intra-arterial cisplatin and doxorubicin were administered at 3-week intervals, with radiotherapy administered for 4 weeks (Mokarim, et al., 1997). This study showed complete response rates and tumor-free bladder preservation rates of 74% and 54%, respectively. Unfortunately, these reports had relatively small numbers of patients (under 50 patients).

At present, chemoradiation therapy incorporating this infusion protocol has resulted in high complete remission (CR) rates of 83%-93% in patients with locally invasive bladder cancer (Miyanaga, et al., 2000; Eapen, et al., 2004; Hashine et al., 2009). These rates seem to be higher than the CR rates of conventional chemoradiation therapies, although a simple comparison is impossible. However, these studies have also shown 5-year overall survival rates of 50%-66.6% (Miyanaga, et al., 2000; Eapen, et al., 2004; Hashine, et al., 2009), which were similar to the results of other studies using intravenous infusion (Table 2). Problems with this strategy include specific complications (pelvic neuropathy and risk of severe bleeding) and the complexity of the procedure. There has been only one report in a large study population on trimodality bladder preservation incorporating intra-arterial chemotherapy (Eapen, et al., 2004).

With regard to this treatment strategy, there has been a unique and interesting trial (Azuma, et al., 2008) of combined therapy using balloon-occluded arterial infusion of CDDP and hemodialysis with concurrent radiation. In this regimen, the study patients underwent TUR and received balloon-occluded arterial infusion of 100-300 mg CDDP, together with concurrent hemodialysis and a total of 60.4 Gy of radiation. In the first report, this therapy had been administered to 41 patients with T2-4NxM0 disease. All patients with transitional cell carcinoma with T2-3 achieved a complete response (n = 29) and were able to retain their bladders with no evidence of recurrence at a mean follow-up of 132 weeks (Azuma, et al., 2008).

4.3. Partial cystectomy in the bladder conservation strategy

With regard to surgery in bladder conservation therapy, TUR has been used in almost all of the large studies (Table 2). On the other hand, several studies used partial cystectomy as the primary therapy in their treatment strategy (Holzbeierlein et al., 2004; Kassouf et al., 2006; Zhang et al., 2010). As mentioned above, radical cystectomy is the "gold standard" for surgical treatment in patients with MIBC. In contrast, partial cystectomy provides a surgical alternative for selected patients because patients who undergo partial cystectomy are considered to be at higher risk for tumor recurrence and the need for second surgery (Evans and Texter, 1975; Stein et al., 2001). Some authors hold the opinion that partial cystectomy is disproportionately used and that overuse of this operation may constitute inappropriate delivery of health care (Hollenbeck, et al., 2005). For these reasons, partial cystectomy is generally the recommended treatment for adenocarcinoma and/or urothelial carcinoma at the dome of the urinary bladder. However, there is no escaping the fact that partial cystectomy has potential advantages compared with radical cystectomy, for example, functional advantages including continence and sexual function, decreased incidence of surgical morbidity, and avoidance of the need for urinary diversion. In recent years, population-based and matched case-control studies have demonstrated that partial and radical cystectomy provided similar oncologic control and outcome, including metastasis-free and cause-specific survival (Capitanio, et al., 2009; Knoedler, et al., 2012). However, the fact remains that these results are obtained in "selected" patients. In fact, two large cancer centers (Memorial Sloan-Kettering Cancer Center and M.D. Anderson Cancer Center) have suggested that stringent selection of appropriate patients improves cancer control rates after partial cystectomy for patients with MIBC (Holzbeierlein, et al., 2004; Kassouf, et al., 2006).

Ideal candidates for partial cystectomy are patients with a solitary tumor located in a resectable area not requiring ureteral re-implantation, such as the dome of the urinary bladder, and which can be resected with a 1-2 cm tumor-free margin to preserve normal bladder function. Patients with associated carcinoma in situ should be excluded. Only 3%-10% of MIBC patients who are candidates for cystectomy fit these criteria (Holzbeierlein, et al., 2004; Kassouf, et al., 2006; Capitanio, et al., 2009). Marked variation in outcome after partial cystectomy has been reported: the 5-year recurrence-free survival rates in separate series from M.D. Anderson Cancer Center and Memorial Sloan-Kettering Cancer Center are 39% and 69%, respectively. The bladder conservation strategy of partial cystectomy requires careful attention to patient selection criteria in order to obtain optimal therapeutic outcome.

In recent years, laparoscopy with or without robotic radical cystectomy has begun to be performed; this technique may lead to less bleeding, less post-operative pain, and earlier recovery (Khan, et al., 2012). However, the long-term outcome is unclear, and the operation requires a longer duration and engenders higher cost compared with open surgery. These remain problems to be solved. Likewise, several studies and the experience of several authors with robotic partial cystectomy have been reported (Luchey, et al., 2012; Seyam, et al., 2012). However, almost all of these procedures have been performed on benign tumors including paraganglioma and lymphangioma. On the other hand, there has been a pilot study of robotic partial cystectomy for bladder cancer (Allaparthi, et al., 2010). Similar to radical cystectomy, obstacles to robotic partial cystectomy are high cost, technical difficulties such as decisions regarding tumor margin, and relatively low numbers of ideal patients. The immediate future and further applications of robotic partial cystectomy for bladder cancer are uncertain.

5. GC regimen in peri-operative therapies

For the last several decades, MVAC and CMV (cisplatin, methotrexate, vinblastine) have been especially employed for treating advanced urothelial carcinoma. Additionally, these regimens have been used in almost all of the trials and studies on peri-operative chemotherapy. On the other hand, the GC regimen has been reported as an alternative regimen and more tolerable than the MVAC/CMV regimen in treating advanced urothelial cancer (von der Maase, et al., 2005). In addition to treating advanced disease, the GC regimen seems more advantageous than the MVAC/CMV regimen because the GC regimen has a lower toxicity profile and therefore reduces the potential need for changing the treatment schedule because of toxic side effects. Actually, various studies on peri-operative therapy with GC regimen have been reported. In recent year, a randomized phase III trial of adjuvant GC therapy in 194 patients with pT2G3-pT4N0-2 disease was reported. This manuscript demonstrated that 5-year overall survival rate in adjuvant therapy (43.4%) was similar (P=0.24) to that in control (observation and treatment on relapse) (53.7%).

On the other hand, several studies on the local therapeutic effects of neo-adjuvant GC therapy have been published (Table 3). In the series by Dash et al., pT0 was detected in 11 of 42 patients receiving the GC regimen (26%) and in 15 of 54 patients receiving the MVAC regimen (28%). From these results, Dash et al. (2008) concluded that the GC regimen has ability similar to that of the MVAC regimen for inducing pathological down-staging in bladder cancer patients with locally advanced disease. Similar results (showing complete response of MVAC = 31% and GC = 25%) were reported in 2012 by Yeshchina et al. On the other hand, Weight, et al. (2009) reported that the percentages of patients presenting with stage pT0 at the time of definitive surgery who were treated with the neo-adjuvant GC regimen or with cystectomy alone were 10% (2/20) and 9% (8/88), respectively. In recent years, larger studies with a similar design showed that pT0 was detected in 20% (5 of 25) of patients with neo-adjuvant CG and 5% (7 of 135 patients) with cystectomy alone (Scosyrev et al., 2011). These authors concluded that the neo-adjuvant GC regimen was capable of down-staging bladder cancer. Interestingly, Scosyrev et al. also suggested that GC has no effect on disease involving the lymph nodes. Unfortunately, these studies were relatively small series and consisted of patients with a variety of clinicopathological features. Furthermore, the long-term outcome after the GC- and GEM-based regimens for peri-operative treatment is still not fully known. Currently, in clinical practice, including phase II trials, a less toxic GC regimen is commonly substituted for peri-operative MVAC therapy.

Author (year)	N	Clinical stage	Induction	pT0 (%)	P value	Comments
Dash (2008)	A: 42 B: 54	T2-4N0M0	A: GC + cystectomy B: MVAC + cystectomy	26 28	–	No difference in down-staging, disease-free survival, or residual disease. .
Weight (2009)	A: 20 B: 88	T2-4aN0-2M0	A: GC+radical cystectomy B: Radical cystectomy only	10 9	–	This study included 20 patients with GC (PTX in 1) and 9 with other regimens. .
Scosyrev (2012)	A: 25 B: 135	T2-4NanyM0	A: GC+radical cystectomy B: Radical cystectomy only	20 5	P=0.03	Capable of down-staging (proportion of pT0), but no effect on disease in node.
Yeshchina (2012)	A: 16 B: 45	T2-4aN0-2M0	A: GC + radical cystectomy B: MAVC + radical cystectomy	25 31	P=0.645	This choice also affected no significant difference in adjuvant therapy (n=53).

Table 3. Neo-adjuvant gemcitabine plus cisplatin for muscle invasive bladder cancer

6. Molecular-targeted therapy in peri-operative therapy

When molecular targeted therapy is performed, understanding of its clinical significance, pathological roles, and prognostic value is essential. We therefore introduce some molecules that are closely associated with malignant potential and aggressiveness in bladder cancer.

Phase	Intervention	Sponsor	Start year	On going	Identifier : NCT-
0	Lapatinib	University Hospital, Bordeaux	2012	Yes	01245660
I	Intravesical vaccine (rF-GM-CSF, -TRICOM)	University of Medicine and Dentistry of New Jersey	2003	No	00072137
II	IFM, DXR, GEM, CDDP	M.D. Anderson Cancer Center	2001	No	00080795
II	MVAC, bevacizmab	M.D. Anderson Cancer Center	2007	Yes	00506155
II	CBDCA, GEM, ABI-007	University of Michigan	2007	Yes	00585689
II	Dose-dense MVAC	Dana-Farber Cancer Institute	2008	Yes	00808639
II	Erotinib	M.D. Anderson Cancer Center	2008	Yes	00749892
II	Sunitinib after cystectomy following prior neo-adjuvant	University of Michigan	2009	Yes	01042795
II	GEM, CDDP, Sunitinib	MSKCC	2009	Yes	00847015
II	Dose-dense MVAC	Fox Chase Cancer Center	2009	Yes	01031420
II	GEM, CDDP, Sunitinib	Hoosier Oncology Group	2008	No	00859339
II	GEM, CDDP, Sorafenib	Fondazione IRCCS Istituto Nazionale dei tumori	2010	Yes	01222676
II	CDDP, cabazitaxel	United Bistrol Healthcare NHS Trust	2012	Yes	01616875
II	Dose-dense GC	MSKCC	2012	Yes	01589094

Table 4. Clinical trials of neo-adjuvant therapies

6.1. p53

p53 regulates the cell cycle through inhibition of the cell cycle progression at the G1/S transition, and p53 is also involved in various important cellular processes related to angiogenesis, DNA repair, apoptosis, and response to therapy in bladder cancer cells (Mitra, et al., 2006). The first report on the prognostic value of p53 expression in patients with bladder cancer demonstrated that p53 expression status predicted recurrence and survival after radical cystectomy in patients with organ-confined bladder cancer (Esrig, et al., 1994). After that, many investigators showed that p53 mutations occur in approximately 50% of cases of bladder cancer, and that altered p53 status is a useful predictor for cancer cell progression and outcome in bladder cancer patients (Sarkis, et al. 1993; Esrig, et al., 1994; Serth, et al., 1995). However, there was controversial opinion regarding the prognostic value of p53. Actually, a meta-analysis that reviewed 117 studies with 10,026 patients showed that there is insufficient evidence to know whether p53 can serve as a prognostic marker for bladder cancer (Malats, et al., 2005).

Two independent clinical trials regarding p53 gene therapy were performed in a phase I study. A study (SCH 58500) of the safety, feasibility, and biological activity of an adenoviral expression vector encoding wild-type p53 was performed in 12 patients with histologically confirmed

MIBC (Kuball, et al., 2002). In another study, replication-deficient adenoviral vectors bearing the wild-type TP53 gene (Ad5CMV-TP53) were transferred into bladder cancer cells of advanced disease by repeated (28-day cycle) intravesical instillation in 13 patients with locally advanced disease (Pagliaro, et al., 2003). These studies showed that such methods are safe, without no dose-limiting toxicity, and feasible for treatment of patients with bladder cancer. Yet, although the use of gene therapy in combination with transduction-enhancing agents increased transduction efficacy and promoted a high level of patient tolerance, some investigators believe that more improvements in the efficacy of gene transfer and greater knowledge of gene expression levels are required to develop more effective gene therapy.

There is the opinion that locally advanced bladder cancer cells that harbor p53 alterations may respond beneficially to adjuvant chemotherapy containing DNA-damaging agents (Cote, et al., 1997). In addition, there have been several reports that DNA-damaging agents such as CDDP can increase the sensitivity of the bladder cancer cell lines (Lai, et al., 2005; Matsui, et al., 2007). Thus, gene therapy that targets p53 alterations has the possibility of being effective for bladder cancer patients with advanced disease.

6.2. Epidermal Growth Factor Receptor (EGFR)

Among the members of the EGFR family, ErbB1 and ErbB2 (Her2/neu) are the most studied in human cancers. There is general agreement that they are overexpressed in the majority of patients with urothelial cancer of the urinary bladder, including MIBC, and are positively associated with pathological features (Wright, et al., 1991; Korkolopoulou, et al., 1997, Kossouf, et al., 2008). Furthermore, with regard to their predictive value for prognosis and survival, increased expression of these two molecules has been reported to be associated with worse outcome (Korkolopoulou, et al., 1997; Krüger, et al. 2002; Kramer, et al., 2007). In addition, overexpression of EGFR is known to be more common in MIBC (Kassouf, et al., 2008). From these facts, there is a possibility that EGFR-targeted therapies have the potential to improve prognosis and survival in patients with MIBC.

On the other hand, there have been several reports that ErbB2 expression is not correlated with any pathological features, including grade and stage or survival, in bladder cancer patients (Jimenez, et al., 2001; Kassouf, et al., 2007). To explain this discrepancy in the research findings, differences in patient backgrounds and evaluation methods have been suggested. The differing reports show that there is no general agreement about the pathological significance and prognostic role of the EGFR in patients with bladder cancer. Jimenez et al. made the interesting observation that the frequencies of overexpression of ErbB2 in primary tumors and in metastatic tumors were 37% and 63%, respectively (Jimenez, et al., 2001). This finding may suggest that ErbB2 could be an effective therapeutic target for the inhibition of cancer cell progression after treatment of primary tumors.

Gefitinib (brand name, Iressa) is a small molecular EGFR tyrosine kinase inhibitor that selectively inhibits EGFR. Several clinical trials with gefitinib are now in progress. The results of Cancer and Leukemia Group B (CALGB) study number 9012 showed 23 confirmed objective responses (7 complete responses and 16 partial responses) in 54 assessable patients. The median time to progression and overall survival were 7.4 months and 15.1 months, respectively. Based on these results, the authors concluded that outcomes and survivals were not significantly superior to those of previously reported results with GC alone (Philips et al., 2009).However, there is a report that response rate and overall survival after combination therapy with gefitinib and GC were similar to the rates using GC therapy alone in 54 chemotherapy-naïve patients with locally advanced and metastatic urothelial cancer (Philips, et al., 2009).

Cetuximab (Erbitux) is an intravenously administered monoclonal antibody against the EGFR. In animal studies, cetuximab showed anti-growth activity against bladder cancer cells (Perrotte, et al., 1999). Furthermore, the combination of paclitaxel and cetuximab exhibited synergistic growth inhibition by suppression of proliferation and enhancement of apoptosis in tumor and endothelial cells in a murine model of metastatic human bladder cancer (Inoue, et al., 2000). Thus, cetuximab is expected to have a remarkable anti-tumor effect in patients with advanced bladder cancer. A study comparing the effects of GC with or without cetuximab in bladder cancer patients with locally advanced or metastatic disease is currently underway in a phase II setting.

Trastuzumab (Herceptin) is a recombinant humanized monoclonal antibody to ErbB2 (HER2). This drug has been reported to be safe and effective in other types of malignancies, especially breast cancer (Burstein, et al., 2003). For treating bladder cancer, a phase II study of the effects of second-line treatment with trastuzumab monotherapy in patients with metastatic urothelial cancer and HER2 overexpression was completed in Germany (protocol number ML17599). In addition, a multicenter phase II trial investigating trastuzumab together with paclitaxel, carboplatin, and gemcitabine was conducted in 57 patients with advanced urothelial cancer having positive expression of ErbB2 as determined by immunohistochemistry (CCUM-9955) (Hussain, et al., 2007). This study showed a 70% response rate, and median times to progression and survival were 9.3 months and 14.1 months, respectively. Interestingly, Trastuzumab is being evaluated in combination with paclitaxel and radiotherapy as a bladder conservation strategy.

Lapatinib is an oral small-molecule dual tyrosine kinase inhibitor of the EGFR and ErbB2. It produces a remarkable response and anti-tumor effect in patients with urothelial cancer. Synergic anti-tumor effects with various chemotherapy regimens are known to occur in urothelial cancer cell lines (McHugh, et al., 2007). This phenomenon may enable reduced-dose chemotherapy and/or reduced toxicity. On the other hand, a phase II study by Wulfing et al. (2005) showed disappointing results in that only 2 out of 59 study patients showed partial response when treated with lapatinib. Further studies and trials are necessary to obtain details with regard to the optimal use and efficacy of lapatinib.

Erlotinib (Tarceva) is an oral small-molecule EGFR tyrosine kinase inhibitor. It has characteristics that inhibit activities of wild-type EGFR and mutant EGFRvIII without decreasing the level of EGFR protein in a reversible manner (Zureikat and McLee, 2008). This agent has been approved for metastatic non-small cell lung cancer and metastatic pancreatic cancer. In bladder cancer, several clinical trials, including a phase II study, are exploring the use of erlotinib as a prevention strategy or as neo-adjuvant therapy (NCT00749892).

6.3. Vasculogenesis-related factors

Bevacizumab (Avastin) is a monoclonal antibody that acts as a VEGF inhibitor. It can bind all VEGF isoforms. Bevacizumab is approved by the FDA for treating various solid tumors, including colorectal cancer, breast cancer, and renal cell carcinoma. In urothelial cancer, a phase II trial is being conducted on the use of cisplatin, gemcitabine and bevacizumab in combination for metastatic urothelial cancer (Cancer: Hoosier Oncology Group, study number GU04-75). A study by Hahn et al. (2011) showed that the best response, according to the Response Evaluation Criteria in Solid Tumors, was complete response in 8 patients (19%) and partial response in 23 patients (53%), out of 43 patients with metastatic or unresectable disease. In addition, it showed that the median progression-free survival was 8.2 months, with a median overall survival time of 19.1 months. Based on these results, these investigators concluded that the full risk and benefit profile of this treatment in patients with metastatic urothelial cancer will be determined by an ongoing phase III trial. In another study, phase II trials are evaluating a neo-adjuvant GC regimen on the use of dose-dense (DD)-MVAC + bevacizumab followed by radical cystectomy in patients with MIBC and patients with resectable urothelial cancer of the bladder (NCT-00506155). An interesting pre-clinical trial involving bevacizumab is being conducted, testing a combination of photodynamic therapy (well-known as an emerging diagnostic and therapeutic strategy in bladder cancer [Patel, et al., 2011]), bevacizumab, and fluorescence confocal endomicroscopy as a promising cancer treatment approach (Bhuvaneswari, et al., 2010). A similar treatment strategy using a combination of photodynamic therapy and molecular targeted therapy is being investigated by another study group using bevaxizmab and cetuximab in a murine bladder cancer model (Bhuvaneswari et al., 2011).

Thrombospondin (TSP)-1 is well-known as a representative molecule having anti-angiogenic properties under physiological and pathological conditions. In bladder cancer, TSP-1 expression has been negatively associated with malignant aggressiveness. (Grossfeld, et al., 2003). This report also showed decreased expression of TSP-1 has been observed to predict poor survival in patients with bladder cancer. Interestingly, these investigators also found that alteration of p53 may decrease TSP-1 expression in bladder cancer. From these results, TSP-1 is speculated to be an effective and potential target for novel therapies. Actually, a plan for TSP-1-target therapy has already been in existence and has been investigated in preclinical studies, including a phase I trial (Taraboletti, et al., 2010; Li, et al., 2011). Unfortunately, such a clinical trial is not being conducted in patients with MIBC.

7. Conclusions

In this paper, we described various trials and newly treatment strategies for patients with MIBC. In present, choice of all or a part of operation, chemotherapy, and radiation therapy is major treatment strategy for these patients. In addition, molecular-targeted therapy will be added to these conventional therapies in near feature. However, many urologist, medical oncologist, and radiation oncologists have a feeling that the near future strategies may not adequate to give satisfaction for outcome and survival in MIBC disease. So, numerous investigators keep on studying the pathological features and molecular mechanism of bladder cancer to break through the difficulty of the present strategies. We hope more detailed basic studies and precise clinical trials in bladder cancer.

Author details

Yasuyoshi Miyata* and Hideki Sakai

*Address all correspondence to: int.doc.miya@m3.dion.ne.jp

Department of Nephro-Urology, Nagasaki University Graduate School of Biomedical Sciences, Sakamoto, Nagasaki, Japan

References

[1] Advanced Bladder Cancer (ABC) Meta-analysis Collaboration. (2003). Neoadjuvant chemotherapy in invasive bladder cancer: a systematic review and meta-analysis of individuals patient data. *Lancet* 361: 1927-1934.

[2] Advanced Bladder Cancer (ABC) Meta-analysis Collaboration. (2005). Neoadjuvant chemotherapy in invasive bladder cancer: update of a systematic review and meta-analysis of individuals patient data. *Eur Urol* 48: 202-206.

[3] Alva, A.S., Tallman, T.T., He, C., Hussain, M.H., Hafez, K., Montie, J.E., Smith, D.C., Weizer, A.Z., Wood, D. & Lee, C.T. (2012). Efficient delivery of radical cystectomy after neoadjuvant chemotherapy for muscle-invasive bladder cancer. A multidisciplinary approach. *Cancer* 118: 44-53.

[4] Allaparthi, S., Ramanathan, R. & Balaji, K.C. (2010). Robotic partial cystectomy for bladder cancer: a single-institutional pilot study. *J Endourol* 24: 223-227.

[5] Azuma, H., Kotake Y., Yamamoto, K., Sakamoto, T., Kiyama, S., Ubai, T., Inamoto, T., Takahara, K., Matuski, M., Segawa, N., et al. (2008). Effect of combined therapy using balloon-occluded arterial infusion of cisplatin and hemodialysis with concurrent radiation for locally invasive bladder cancer. *Am J Clin Oncol* 31: 11-21.

[6] Bhuvaneswari, R., Thong, P.S., Gan, Y.Y., Soo, K.C. & Olivo, M. (2010). Evaluation of hypericin-mediated photodynamic therapy in combination with angiogenesis inhibitor bevacizumab using in vivo fluorescence confocal endomicroscopy. *J Biomed Opt* 15: 011114

[7] Bhuvaneswari, R., Yuen, G.Y., Chee, S.K. & Olivo, M. (2010). Antiangiogenic agents avastin and Erbitux enhance the efficacy of photodynamic therapy in amurin bladder tumor model. *Laser Surg Med* 43: 651-662.

[8] Burstein, H.J., Harris, L.N., Marcom, P.K., Lambert-Falls, R., Havlin, K., Overmoyer, B., Friedlander, R.J. Jr., Gargiulo, J., Strenger, R., Vogel, C.L., Ryan, P.D., et al. (2003). Trastuzumab and vinorelbine as first-line therapy for HER2-overexpressing metastatic breast cancer: multicenter phase II trial with clinical outcomes, analysis of serum tumor markers as predictive factors, and cardiac surveillance algorithm. J Clin Oncol 21: 2889-2895.

[9] Calabro, F & Sternberg, CN. (2009) Neoadjuvant and adjuvant chemotherapy in muscle-invasive bladder cancer. *Eur Urol* 55: 348-358.

[10] Capitanio, U., Isbarn, H., Shariat, S.F., Jeldres, C., Zini, L., Saad, F., Graefen, M., Montorsi, F., Perrotte, P. & Karakiewicz, P.I. (2009). Partial cyctectomy does not undermine cancer control in appropriate selected patients with urothelial carcinoma of the bladder: a population-based matched analysis. *Urology* 74: 858-864.

[11] Chen, L., Agrawal, S., Zhou, W., Zhang, R. & Chen, J. (1998). Synergistic activation of p53 by inhibition of MDM2 expression and DNA damage. *Proc Natl Acad Sci U S A* 95: 195-200.

[12] Cognetti, F., Ruggeri, E.M., Felici, A., Galluci, M., Muto, G., Pollera, C.F., Massidda, B., Rubagotti, A., Giannarelli, D. & Boccardo, F. (2012). on behalf of the Study Group. Adjuvant chemotherapy with cisplatin and gemcitabine versus chemotherapy at relapse in patients with muscle-invasive bladder cancer submitted to radical cystectomy: an Italian, multicenter, randomized phase III trial. *Ann Oncol* 23: 695-700.

[13] Cote, R.J., Esrig, D., Groshen, S., Jones, PA. & Skinner, D.G. (1997). p53 and treatment of bladder cancer. *Nature* 385: 123-125.

[14] Dash, A., Pettus, J.A, 4th., Herr, H.W., Borchnerm B.H., Dallbagni, G., Donat, S.M., Russo, P., Boyle, M.G., Milowsky, M.I. & Bajorin, D.F. (2008). A role of neoadjuvant gemicitabine plus cisplatin in muscle-invasive urothelial carcinoma of the bladder. *Cancer* 113: 2471-2477.

[15] Donat SM, Shabsigh A, Savage C, Cronin, A.M., Bochner, B.H., Dalbagni, G., Herr, H.W. & Milowsky, M.I. (2009). Potential impact of postoperative early complication on the timing of adjuvant chemotherapy in patients undergoing radical cystectomy: a high-volume tertiary cancer center experience. *Eur Urol* 55: 177-186.

[16] Eapen, L., Stewart, D., Collins, J. & Peterson, R. (2004). Effective bladder sparing therapy with intra-arterial cisplatin and radiotherapy for localized bladder cancer. *J Urol* 172: 1276-1280.

[17] Efstathiou, J.A., Spiegel, D.Y., Shipley, W.U., Heney, N.M., Kaufman, D.S., Niemierko, A., Coen, J.J., Skowronski, T.Y., Paly, J.J., McGovern, F.J., *et al.* (2012). Long-term

outcomes of selective bladder preservation by combined-modality therapy for invasive bladder cancer: the MGH experience. *Eur Urol* 61: 705-711.

[18] Esrig, D., Elmajian, D., Groshen, S., Freeman, J.A., Stein, J.P., Chen, S.C., Nichols, P.W., Skinner, D.G., Jones, P.A. & Cote, R.J. Accumulation of nuclear p53 and tumor progression in bladder cancer. *N Engl J Med* 331: 1259-1264.

[19] Evans, R.A. & Texter, J.H. (1975). Partial cyctectomy in treatment of bladder cancer. *J Urol* 114: 391-393.

[20] Feifer, A., Tayor, J.M., Shouery, M., Steinberg, G.D., Stadler, W.M., Schoenberg, M., Zlotta, A., Lerner, S.P., Bajorin, D.F. & Bochner, B. (2011). Multi-institutional quality-of-care initiative for nonmetastatic, muscle-invasive, transitional cell carcinoma of the bladder [abstract 240]. *J Clin Oncol* ; 29 (Supple 7).

[21] Gamal El-deen, H., Elshazly, H.F. & Abo Zeina, E.A. (2009). Clinical experience with radiotherapy alone and radiochemotherapy with platin based regimens in organ-sparing treatment of invasive bladder cancer. *J Egypt Natl Cancer Inst* 21: 59-70.

[22] Ghoneim, M.A., Abdel-Latif, M., el-Mekresh, M., Abol-Enein, H., Mosbah, A., Ashamallah, A. & wl-Baz, M.A. (2008). Radical cystectomy for carcinoma of the bladder: 2720 consecutive cases 5 years later. *J Urol* 180: 121-127.

[23] Goethuys, H. and Van Poppel, H. (2012). Update on management of invasive bladder cancer 2012. *Cancer Manag Res* 4: 177-182.

[24] Griffiths, G., Hall, R., Sylvester, R., Raghavan, D. & Parmar, M.K. (2011). International pahse III trials assessing neoadjuvant cisplatin, methotrexate, and vinblastine chemotherapy for muscle-invasive bladder cancer: long-term results of BA06 30894 trial. *J Clin Oncol* 29: 2171-2177.

[25] Grossfeld, G.D., Ginsberg, D.A., Stein, J.P., Bochner, B.H., Esrig, D., Groshen, S., Dunn, M., Nichols, P.W., Taylor, C.R., Skinner, D.G., et al. (1997). Thrombospondin-1 expression in bladder cancer: association with p53 alterations, tumor angiogenesis, and tumor progression. *J Natl Cancer Inst*. 89: 219-227.

[26] Grossman, H.B., Natale, R.B., Tangen, C.M., Speights, V.O., Vogelzang, N.J., Trump, D.L., deVere White, R.W., Sarosdy, M.F., Wood, D.P. Jr., Raghavan, D. & Crawford, ED. (2003). Neoadjuvant chemotherapy plus cystectomy compared with cystectomy alone for locally advanced bladder cancer. *N Engl J Med* 349: 859-866.

[27] Hahn, N.M., Stadler, W.M., Zon, R.T., Waterghouse, D., Picus, J., Nattam, S., Johnson, C.S., Perkins, S.M., Waddell, M.J. & Sweeney, C.J. (2011). Pahse II trila of cisplatin, gemcitabine, and bevacizumab as first-line therapy for metastatic urothelial carcinoma: Hossier Oncology Group GU 04-75. *J Clin Oncol* 29: 1525- 1530.

[28] Hashine, K., Kusuhara, Y., Miura, N., Shirato, A., Sumiyoshi, Y., & Kataoka, M. (2009). Bladder prevention therapy conducted by intra-arterial chemotherapy and radiotherapy for muscle invasive bladder cancer. *Jpn J Clin Oncol* 39: 381-386.

[29] Herr, H.W., Bajorin, D.F. & Scher, H.I. (1998). Neoadjuvant chemotherapy and bladder-sparing surgery for invasive bladder cancer: ten-year outcome. *J Clin Oncol* 16: 1298-1301.

[30] Hollenbeck, B.K., Taub, D.A., Dunn, R.L. & Wei, J.T. (2005). Quality of care: partial cystectomy for bladder cancer—a case of inappropriate use? *J Urol* 174: 1050-1054.

[31] Holzbeierlein, J.M., Lopez-Corona, E., Bochner, B.H., Herr, H.W., Donat, S.M., Russo, P., Dallbagni, G. & Sogani, P.C. (2004). Partial cystectomy: a contemporary review of the Memorial Sloan-Kettering Cancer Center experience and recommendations for patient selection. *J Urol* 172: 878-881.

[32] Housset, M., Maulard, C., Chretien, Y., Dufour, B., Delanian, S., Huart, J., Colardelle, F., Brunel, P. & Baillet F. (1993). Combined radiation and chemotherapy for invasive transitional-cell carcinoma of the bladder: a prospective study. *J Clin Oncol* 11: 2150-2157.

[33] Hussain, S.A. and James, N.D. (2003). The systemic treatment of advanced and metastatic bladder cancer. *Lancet Oncol* 4: 489-497.

[34] Hussain, M.H., MacVicar, G.R., Petrylak, D.P., Dunn, R.L., Vaishampayan, U., Lara, P.N. Jr., Chatta, G.S., Nanus, D.M., Glode, L.M., Trump, D.L., *et al.*(2007) National Cancer Institute. Trastuzumab, paclitaxel, carboplatin, and gemcitabine in advanced human epidermal growth factor receptor-2/neu-positive urothelial carcinoma: results of a multicenter phase II National Cancer Institute trial. *J Clin Oncol* 25: 2218-2224.

[35] Inoue, K., Slaton, J.W., Perrotte, P., Davis, D.W., Bruns, C.J., Hicklin, D.J., McConkey, D.J., Sweeney, P., Radinsky, R. & Dinney CP. (2000). Paclitaxel enhances the effects of the antiepidermal growth factor receptor monoclonal antibody ImVlone C225 in mice with metastatic human bladder transitional cell carcinoma. *Clin Cancer Res* 6: 4874-4884.

[36] International collaboration of trialists. (1999). Neoadjuvant cisplatin, methotrexate, and vinblastine chemotherapy for muscle-invasive bladder cancer: a randomised controlled trial. International collaboration of trialists. *Lancet* 354: 533-540.

[37] International Collaboration of Trialists. (2011). International phase III trial assessing neoadjuvant cisplatin, methotrexate, and vinblastine chemotherapy for muscle-invasive bladder cancer: long-term results of the BA06 30894 trial. *J Clin Oncol* 29: 2171-2177.

[38] Jimenez, R.E., Hussain, M., Bianco, F.J. Jr., Vaishampayan, U., Tabazcka, P., Sakr, W.A., Pontes, J.E., Wood, D.P. Jr. & Grignon, D.J. (2001). Her-2/neu overexpression in muscle-invasive urothelial carcinoma of the bladder: prognostic significance and comparative analysis in primary and metastatic tumors. *Clin Cancer Res* 7: 2440-2447.

[39] Kachnic, L.A., Kaufman, D.S., Heney, N.M., Althausen, A.F., Griffin, P.P., Zietman, A.L. & Shipley, W.U. (1997). Bladder preservation by combined modality therapy for invasive bladder cancer. *J Clin Oncol* 15: 1022-1029.

[40] Kassouf, W., Swanson, D., Kamat, A.M., Leibovici, D., Siefker-Radtke, A., Munsell, M.F., Grossman, H.B. & Dinney, C.P. (2006). Partial cystectomy for muscle invasive urothelial carcinoma of the bladder: a contemporary review of the M. D. Anderson Cancer Center experience. *J Urol* 175: 2058-2062.

[41] Kassouf, W., Black, P.C., Tuziak, T., Bondaruk, J., Lee, S., Brown, G.A., Adam, L., Wei, C., Baggerly, K., Bar-Eli, M. *et al.* (2008). Distinctive expression pattern of ErbB family receptors signifies an aggressive variant of bladder cancer. *J Urol* 179: 353-358.

[42] Kaufman, D.S., Shipley, W.U., Griffin, P.P., Heney, N.M., Althausen, A.F. & Efird, J.T. (1993). Selective bladder preservation by combination treatment of invasive bladder cancer. *N Engl J Med* 4: 1377-1382.

[43] Kaufman, D.S., Shipley, W.U. & Feldman, A.S. (2009). Bladder cancer. *Lancet* 374: 239-249.

[44] Kaufman, D.S., Winter, K.A., Shipley, W.U., Heney, N.M., Wallace III, H.J., Toonkel, L.M., Zietman, A.L., Tanguay, S. & sandler H.M. (2009). Phase I-II RTOG study (99-06) of patients with muscle-invasive bladder cancer undergoing transurethral surgery, paclitaxel, cisplatin, and twice-daily radiotherapy followed by selective bladder preservation or radical cystectomy and adjuvant chemotherapy. *Urology* 73: 833-837.

[45] Khan, M.S., Challacombe, B., Elhage, O., Rimington, P., Coker, B., Murphy, D., Grieve, A. & Dasgupta P. (2012). A dual-centre, cohort comparison of open laparoscopic and robotic-associated radical cystectomy. *Int J Clin Pract*, in press.

[46] Knoedler, J.J., Boorjian, S.A., Kim, B.S., Weight, C.J., Thapa, P., Tarrell, R.F., Cheville, J.C. & frank, I. (2012). Does partial cystectomy compromise oncologic outcomes for patients with bladder cancer compared to radical cystectomy? A matched case-control analysis. *J Urol*, in press.

[47] Korkolopoulou, P., Christodoulou, P., Kapralos, P., Exarchakos, M., Bisbiroula, A., Hadjiyannakis, M., Georgountzos, C. & Thomas-Tsagli, E. (1997) The role of p53, MDM2 and c-erb B-2 oncoproteins, epidermal growth factor receptor and proliferation markers in the prognosis of urinary bladder cancer. Pathol Res Pract 193, 767-775.

[48] Kramer, C., Klasmeyer, K., Bojar, H., Schulz, W.A., Ackermann, R. & Grimm, M.O. (2007). Heparin-binding epidermal growth factor-like growth factor isoforms and epidermal growth factor receptor/ErbB1 expression in bladder cancer and their relation to clinical outcome. *Cancer* 109: 2016-2024.

[49] Krüger, S., Weitsch, G., Büttner, H., Matthiensen, A., Böhmer, T., Marquardt, T., Sayk, F., Feller, A.C. & Böhle, A. (2002). HER2 overexpression in muscle-invasive urothelial carcinoma of the bladder: prognostic implications. *Int J Cancer* 102: 514-518.

[50] Kuball, J., Wen, S.F., Leissner, J., Atkins, D., Meinhardt, .P, Quijano, E., Engler, H., Hutchins, B, Maneval, D.C., Grace, M.J., *et al.* (2002). Successful adenovirus-mediated wild-type p53 gene transfer in patients with bladder cancer by intravesical vector instillation. *J Clin Oncol.* 20:957-965.

[51] Lai, M.D., Lin, W.C., Sun, Y.M. & Chang, F.L. (2005). Phosphorylated and hypoacetylated mutant p53 enhances cisplatin-induced apoptosis through caspase-9 pathway in the absence of transcriptional activation or translation. *Int J Mol Med* 15: 725-734.

[52] Li, L., Leedom, T.A., Do, J., Huang, H., Lai, J.Y., Johnson, K., Osothprarop, T.F., Rizzo, J.D., Doppalapudi, V.R., Bradshaw, C.W., et al. (2011). Antitumoral efficacy of a thrombospondin 1 mimetic CovX-Body. *Trans Oncol* 4: 249-257.

[53] Lunchey, A., Zaslau, S. & Talug C. (2012). Robotic assisted partial cystectomy with pelvic lymph node dissection for metastatic paraganglioma of the urinary bladder. *Can J Urol 19*: 6389-6391.

[54] Malats, N., Bustos, A., Nascimento, C.M., Fernandez, F., Rivas, M., Puente, D., Kogevinas, M. & Real, F.X. (2005). P53 as a prognostic marker for bladder cancer: a meta-analysis and review. Lancet Oncol 6: 678-686.

[55] Malmström, P.U., Rintala, E., Wahlqvist, R., Hellström, P., Hellsten, S. & Hannisdal, E. (1996). Five-year followup of a prospective trial of radical cystectomy and neoadjuvant chemotherapy: Nordic Cystectomy Trial I. The Nordic Cooperative Bladder Cancer Study Group. *J Urol* 155: 1903-1906.

[56] Martinez-Piñeiro, J.A., Gonzalez Martin, M., Arocena, F., Flores, N., Roncero, C.R., Portillo, J.A., Escudero, A., Jimenez Cruz, F. & Isorna, S. (1995). Neoadjuvant cisplatin chemotherapy before radical cystectomy in invasive transitional cell carcinoma of the bladder: prospective randomized phase III study. *J Urol* 153: 964-973.

[57] Manoharan, M., Ayyathurai, R., & Soloway, M.S. (2009). Radical cystectomy for urothelial carcinoma of the bladder: an analysis of perioperative and survival outcome. BJU Int 104: 1227-1232.

[58] Matsui, Y., Ueda, S., Watanabe, J., Kuwabara, I., Ogawa, O. & Nishiyama, H. (2007). Sensitizing effect of galectin-7 in urothelial cancer to cisplatin through the accumulation of intracellular reactive oxygen species. *Cancer Res* 67: 1212-1220.

[59] McHugh, L.A., Kriajevska, M., Mellon, J.K. & Griffiths, T.R. (2007). Combined treatment of bladder cancer cell lines with lapatinib and varying chemotherapy regimens–evidence of schedule-dependent synergy. *Urology* 69: 390-394.

[60] Medical Research Council. (1999). Neoadjuvant cisplatin, methotrexate, and vinblastine chemotherapy for muscle-invasive bladder cancer: a randomized controlled trial. International collaboration of trialists. *Lancet* 354: 533-540.

[61] Messing, E.M., Young, T.B., Hunt, V.B., Gilchrist, K.M., Newton, M.A., Bram, L.L., Hisgen, W.J., Greenberg, E.B., Kuglitsch, M.E. & Wegenke, J.D. (1995). Comparison of bladder cancer outcome in men undergoing hematuria home screening versus those with standard clinical presentation. *Urology* 45: 387-396.

[62] Mitra, A.P., Lin, H., Derar, R.H. & Cote, R.J. (2006). Molecular biology of bladder cancer: prognostic and clinical implications. Clin Genitourin Cancer 5: 67-77.

[63] Miyanaga, N., Akaza, H., Okumura, T., Sekido, N., Kawai, K., Kikuchi, K., Uchida K., Takeshita, H., Ohara, K., Akine, Y., *et al.* (2000). A bladder preservation regimen using intra-arterial chemotherapy and radiotherapy for invasive bladder cancer: a prospective study. *Int J Urol* 7, 41-48.

[64] Mokarim, A., Uetani, M., Hayashi, N., Sakamoto, I., Minami, K., Ogawa, Y., Ochi, M., Matsuoka, Y., Hayashi, K. & Nomata, K . (1997). Combined intraarterial chemotherapy and radiotherapy in the treatment of bladder carcinoma. Cancer 80: 1776-1785.

[65] Pagliaro, L.C., Keyhani, A., Williams, D., Woods, D., Liu, B., Perrotte, P., Slaton, J.W., Merritt, J.A., Grossman, H.B. & Dinney, C.P. (2003). Repeated intravesical instillations of an adenoviral vector in patients with locally advanced bladder cancer: a phase I study of p53 gene therapy. *J Clin Oncol* 22: 2247-2253.

[66] Paramasivan, S., Huddart, R., Hall, E., Lewis, R., Birtle, A. & Donovan, J.L. (2011). Key issues in recruitment to randomized controlled trials with very different interventions: a qualitative investigation of recruitment to the SPARE trial. *Trials* 12: 78

[67] Patel, P., Bryan, R.T. & Wallace, D.M. (2011) Emerging endoscopic and photodynamic technique for bladder cancer detection and surveillance. *ScientificWorldJournal* 11: 2550-2558.

[68] Paz-Ares, L., Solsona, E., Esteban, E., Saez, A., Gonzalez-Larriba, J., Anton, A., Hevia, M., de la Rosa, F., Guillem, V. & Bellmunt, J. (2010). Randomized phase III trial comparing adjuvant paclitaxel/gemcitabine/cisplatin (PCG) to observation in patients with resected invasive bladder cancer: results of the Spanish Oncology Genitourinary Group (SOGUG) 99/01 study (abstract LBA4518). *J Clin Oncol* 28(Suppl): 18s

[69] Perdoná, S., Autorino, R., Damiano, R., De Sio, M., Morrica, B., Gallo, L., Silvestro, G., Farella, A., De Placido, S. & Di Lorenzo, G. (2008). Bladder-sparing, combined approach for muscle-invasive bladder cancer: a multi-institutional, long term experience. *Cancer* 112: 75-83.

[70] Perrotte, P., Matsumoto, T., Inoue, K., Kuniyasu, H., Eve, B.Y., Hicklin, D.J., Radinsky, R. & Dinney, C.P. (1999). Anti-epidermal growth factor receptor antibody C225

inhibits angiogenesis in human transitional cell carcinoma growing orthotopically in nude mice. *Clin Cancer Res* 5: 257-265.

[71] Philips, G.K., Halabi, S., Sanford, B.L., Bajorin, D. & Small, E.J. for the Cancer and Leukemia Goup B. (2009). A phase II trial of cisplatin (C), gemcitabine (G) and gefitinib for advanced urothelial tract carcinoma: results of Cancer and Leukemia Goup B (GALGB) 90102. *Ann Oncol* 20: 1074-1079.

[72] Rogers, C.G., Palapattu, G.S., Shariat, S.F., Karakiewicz, P.I., Bastian, P.J., Lotan, Y., Gupta, A., Vazina, A., Gilad, A., Sagalowsky, A.I., et al. (2006). Clinical outcomes following radical cystectomy for primary nontransitional cell carcinoma of the bladder compared to transitional cell carcinoma of the bladder. *J Urol* 175: 2048-2053.

[73] Rödel, C., Grabenbauer, G.G., Kühn, R., Papadopoulos, T., Dunst, J., Meyer, M., Schrott, K.M. & Sauer, R. (2002). Combined-modality treatment and selective organ presentation in invasive bladder cancer: long-term results. *J Clin Oncol* 20: 3061-3071.

[74] Rosenblatt, R., Sherif, A., Rintala, E., Wahlqvist, R., Ullén, A., Nilsson, S., Pre-Uno, M, the Nordic Urothelial Cancer Group. (2012) Pathologic downstaging is a surrogate marker for efficacy and increased survival following neoadjuvant chemotherapy and radical cystectomy for muscle-invasive urothelial bladder cancer. *Eur Urol* 61: 1229-1238.

[75] Sarkis, A.S., Dalbagni, G., Cordon-Cardo, C., Zhang, Z.F., Sheinfeld, J., Fair, W.R., Herr, H.W. & Reuter, V.E. (1993) Nuclear overexpression of p53 protein in transitional cell bladder carcinoma: a marker for disease progression. *J Natl Cancer Inst* 85:53-59.

[76] Scosyrev, E., Messing, E.M., van Wijngaarden, E., Peterson, D.R., Sahasrabudhe, D., Golijanin, D. & Fisher, S.G. Retrospective analysis of survival in muscle-invasive bladder cancer: impact of pT classification, node status, lymphovascular invasion, and neoadjuvant chemotherapy. *Virchows Arch*, in press.

[77] Serth, J., Kuczyk, M.A., Bokemeyer, C., Hervatin, C., Nafe, R., Tan, H.K. & Jonas U. (1995). p53 immunohistochemistry as an independent prognostic factor for superficial transitional cell carcinoma of the bladder. *Br J Cancer* 71:201-205.

[78] Seyam, R., Alzahrani, H.M., Alkhudair, W.K., Dababo, M.A. & Alotaibi, M.F. (2012). Robotic partial cystectomy for lymphangioma of the urinary bladder in an adult woman. *Can Urol Assoc J* 6: E8-E10.

[79] Shansigh, A., Korets, R., Vora, K.C, Brooks, C.M., Cronin, A.M., Savage, C., Rai, G., Bochner, B.H., Dalbagni, G., Herr, H.W. & Donat, S.M. (2009). Defining eraly morbidity of radical cystectomy for patients with bladder cancer using a standardized reporting methodology. Eur Urol 55: 164-174.

[80] Shariat, F., Karakiewicz, P.I., Palapattu, G.S., Lotan, Y., Rogers, C.G., Amiel, G.E., Vazina, A., Gupta, A., Bastian, P.J., Sagalowsky, A.I. (2006). Outcomes of radical cystec-

tomy for transitional cell carcinoma of the bladder: a contemporary series from the Bladder Cancer Research Consorium. *J Urol* 176: 2414-2422.

[81] Sherif, A., Rintala, E., Mestad, O., Nilsson, J., Holmberg, L., Nilsson, S., Malmström, P.U.; Nordic Urothelial Cancer Group. (2002). Neoadjuvant cisplatin-methotrexate chemotherapy for invasive bladder cancer–Nordic cystectomy trial 2. *Scand J Urol Nephrol* 36: 419-425.

[82] Sherif, A., Holmberg, L., Rintala, E., Mestad, O., Nilsson, J., Nilsson, S., Malmström, P-U; Nordic Urothelial Cancer Group. (2004). Neoadjuvant cisplatinum based combination chemotherapy in patients with invasive bladder cancer: a combined analysis of two Nordic studies. *Eur Urol* 45: 297-303.

[83] Shipley WU, Winter KA, Kaufman DS, Lee, W.R., Heney, N.M., Tester, W.R., Donnelly, B.J., Venner, P.M., Perez, C.A., Murray, K.J., *et al.* (1998). Phase III trial of neoadjuvant chemotherapy in patients with invasive bladder cancer treated with selective bladder preservation by combined radiation therapy and chemotherapy: initial results of Radiation Therapy Oncology Group 89-03. *J Clin Oncol* 16: 3576-3583.

[84] Skinner, D.C., Daniels, J.R., Russell, C.A., Lieskovsky, G., Boyd, S.D., Nichols, P., Kern, W., Sakamoto, J., Krailo, M. & Groshen, S. (1991). The role of adjuvant chemotherapy following cystectomy for invasive bladder cancer: a prospective comparative trial. *J Urol* 145: 459-464.

[85] Stadler, W.M., Lerner, S.P., Groshen, S., Stein, J.P., Shi, S.R., Raghavan, D., Esrig, D., Steinberg, G., Wood, D., Klotz, L., *et al.* (2011). Phase III study of molecularly targeted adjuvant therapy in locally advanced urothelial cancer of the bladder based on p53 status. *J Clin Oncol* 2011; 29: 3443-3449.

[86] Stein, JP., Lieskovsky, G., Cote, R., Groshen, S., Feng, A.C., Boyd, S., Skinner, E., Bochner, B., Thangathurai, D., Mikhail, M., *et al.* (2001) Radical cystectomy in the treatment of invasive bladder cancer: long-term results in 1,054 patients. *J Clin Oncol* 19: 666-675.

[87] Stöckle, M., Meyenburg, W., Wellek, S., Voges, G.E., Rossmann, M., Gertenbach, U., Thüroff, J.W., Huber, C. & Hohenfellner, R. (1995). Adjuvant chemotherapy of nonorgan-confined bladder cancer after radical cyctectomy revisited: long-term results of a controlled prospective study and further clinical experience. *J Urol* 153: 47-52.

[88] Svatek, R.S., Shariat, S.F., Lasky, R.E., Skinner, E.C., Novara, G., Lerner, S.P., Fradet, Y., Bastian, P.J., Kassouf, W., Karakiewicz, P.I., *et al.* (2010). The effectiveness of off-protocol adjuvant chemotherapy for patients with urothelial carcinoma of the urinary bladder. *Clin Cancer Res* 16: 4461-4467.

[89] Taraboletti, G., Rusnati, M., Ragona, L. & Colombo, G. (2010) Targeting tumor angiogenesis with TSP-1-based compounds: rational design of antiangiogenic mimetics of endogenous inhibitors. Oncotarget 1: 662-673.

[90] Von der Maase, H., Sengelov, L., Roberts, J.T., Ricci, S., Dogliotti, L., Oliver, T., Moore, M.J., Zimmermann, A., Arning, M., et al. (2005). Long-term survival results of a randomized trial comparing gemcitabine plus cisplatin, with methotrexate, vinblastine, doxorubicin, plus cisplatin in patients with bladder cancer. *J Clin Oncol* 23: 4602-4608.

[91] Wallace, D.M., Raghavan, D., Kelly, K.A., Sademan, T.F., Conn, I.G., Teriana, N., Dunn, J., Boulas, J. & Latief, T. (1991) Neo-adjuvant (pre-emptive) cisplatin therapy in invasive transitional cell carcinoma. *Br J Urol* 67: 608-615.

[92] Weight, C.J., Garcia, J.A., Hansel, D.E., Fergany, A.F., Campbell, S.C., Gong, M.C., Jones, J.S., Klein, E.A., Dreicer, R. & Stephenson, A.J. (2009). Lack of pathologic down-staging with neoadjuvant chemotherapy for muscle invasive urothelial carcinoma of the bladder. *Cancer* 115: 792-799.

[93] Weiss, S., Engehausen, D.G., Krauses, F.S., Papadopoulos, T., Dunst, J., Sauer, R. & Rödel, C. (2007). Radiochemotherapy with cisplatin and 5-fluorouracil after transurethral surgery in patients with bladder cancer. *Int J Radiat Oncol Biol Phys* 68: 1072-1080.

[94] Winquist, E., Kirchner, T.S., Segal, R., Chin, J. & Lukka, H. (2004). Neoadjuvant chemotherapy for transitional cell carcinoma of the bladder: a systematic review and meta-analysis. *J Urol* 171: 561-569.

[95] Wright, C., Mellon, K., Johnston, P., Lane, D.P., Harris, A.L., Horne, C.H. & Neal, D.E. (1991). Expression of mutant p53, c-erbB-2 and the epidermal growth factor receptor in transitional cell carcinoma of the human urinary bladder. Br J Cancer 63: 967-970.

[96] Wulfing, C., Machiels, J.P., Richel, D., Grimm, M., Treiber, U., de Groot, M., Beuzebec, P., Farrell, J., Stone, N.L., Leopold, L., et al. (2005). A single arm, multicenter, open label, ph II study of lapatinib as 2L treatment of pts with locally advanced/ metastatic transitional cell carcinoma (TCC) of the urothelial tract. *Proc Am Soc Clin Oncol* 23: 16S. Abstarct 4594.

[97] Yeshchina, O., Badalato, G.M., Wosnitzer, M.S., Hruby, G., RoyChoudhury, A., Benson, M.C., Petrylak, D.P. & McKiernan, J.M. (2012). Relative efficacy of perioperative gemcitabine and cisplatin versus methotrexate, vinblastine, Adriamycin, and cisplatin in the management of locally advanced urothelial carcinoma of the bladder. *Urology* 79: 384-390.

[98] Zietman, A.L., Sacco, D., Skowronski, U., Gomery, P., Kaufman, D.S., Clark, J.A., Talcott, J.A., Shipley, W.U. (2003). Transurethral resection, chemotherapy and radiation: results of a urodynamic

[99] and quality of life study on long-term survivors. *J Urol* 170: 1772-1776.

[100] Zietman, A.L., Grocela, J., Zehr, E., Kaufman, D.S., Young, R.H., Althausen, A.F., Heney, N.M. & Shipley, W.U. (2001). Selective bladder conservation using transurethral

resection, chemotherapy, and radiation: management and consequences of Ta, T1 and Tis recurrent within thc related bladder. *Urology* 58: 380-385.

[101] Zureikat, A.H. & McKee, M.D. (2008). Targeted therapy for solid tumors: current status. *Surg Oncol Clin N Am* 17: 279-301, vii-viii.